OTHER WORKS BY
REBECCA SMITH ORLEANE

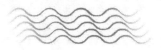

Conversations With Laarkmaa:
A Plieadian View of the New Reality
Co-Author, Cullen Baird Smith

Southern Piercings

DR. REBECCA ORLEANE

THE RETURN
OF THE
feminine

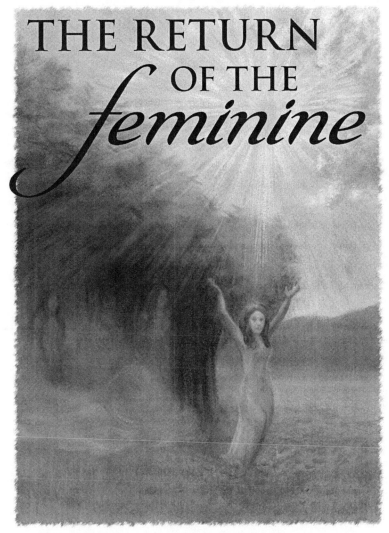

HONORING THE CYCLES OF NATURE

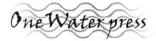 IN
ASSOCIATION
WITH

AuthorHouse™
1663 Liberty Drive
Bloomington, IN 47403
www.authorhouse.com
1-800-839-8640

The information contained in this book is intended to educate, delight, and expand your understanding. It is not intended to diagnose or treat any medical condition, nor is it intended as medical advice. If you have concerns about your health, please consult with a healthcare professional.

Hard cover and soft cover first published by AuthorHouse in association with One Water Press™, 5/28/2010.

ISBN: 978-1-4520-1252-0 (e)
ISBN: 978-1-4520-1250-6 (sc)
ISBN: 978-1-4520-1251-3 (hc)

Library of Congress Control Number: 2010907350

Printed
Bloomington, Indiana, United States of America
This book is printed on acid free paper

Cover:
Art by Ann DiSalvo
Graphic design by Rowan Design

DEDICATION

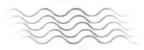

To all those who are remembering the principles
of the Divine Feminine
and are turning towards Nature
to bring balance, harmony, peace, and love to our world.

COVER ART

Ann DiSalvo

INTERIOR PLATES

INTRODUCTION: May Jo Wootten

CHAPTER 1: Donna Hertz

CHAPTER 2: Silvia Trujillo

CHAPTER 3: Paula Fong

CHAPTER 4: Donna Hertz

CHAPTER 5: Paula Fong

CHAPTER 6: Meredith Killmer Hanson

CHAPTER 7: May Jo Wootten

CHAPTER 8: Laura Hurst

CHAPTER 9: Ann DiSalvo

CHAPTER 10: Silvia Trujillo

CHAPTER 11: Paula Fong

CHAPTER 12: Donna Hertz

CHAPTER 13: Silvia Trujillo

EPILOGUE: May Jo Wootten

ART DESIGN AND TYPOGRAPHY

Rowan Design

THE RETURN OF THE FEMININE:
Honoring the Cycles of Nature

Table of Contents

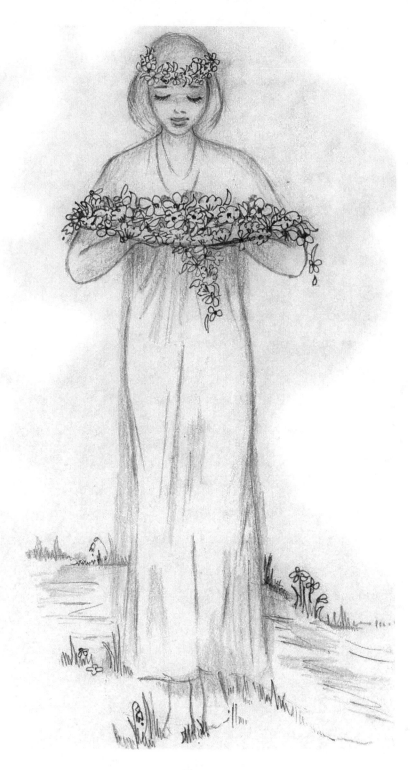

INTRODUCTION

Like all of us, I came from the stars into the rhythms and cycles of Earth. We are Nature beings who are divinely connected to Mother Earth. When I was born I whispered to my mother that I must follow the rhythms of Nature. Listening intently, my mother silently took me to her breast and provided my first cycle of nourishment: her love.

Like so many who are reading this book, I grew up as a young girl in a patriarchal culture. Because of the prevailing attitudes and beliefs, I "lost" (forgot about) my connection to Nature's cycles. I joined the belief system that dictated that "progress" and "linear thinking" were the only systems worthy of recognition. But ignoring my own inner rhythms because they were "inconvenient" or hiding my cycles because they were "embarrassing" and made me "different" from mainstream male culture didn't work for me. I grew pale and sick, unable to be myself.

One day, sitting by the beach and watching the waves come and go, beckoning me to join my water to theirs, I thought to myself, "I am a sun worshiper," as I enjoyed the sun's warmth on my skin. And a voice somewhere in my memory, a voice from the night I arrived on this earth, whispered, "Remember, remember." In an instant, I remembered that I am connected to the sea and the tides. The rhythm of the lapping waves awakened in me the memory of the divinity of my own rhythms: the sea and I were one. I realized that I am connected to and part of Nature, and there can be nothing more holy than the divine cycles which connect us to who we are.

We are 70-98% water. The same salt water that fills the sea fills my blood. The rivers within me are connected to the rivers of Earth. Sitting in the sun, I realized that the energy of the sun not only shines directly on us, but is also reflected from the moon, causing a tidal pull of the water on our planet. As the sea and I are one, my own waters also follow a rhythm of natural cycles. These natural rhythms must be followed to bring our relationships back into balance. This book explores the cycles that define our lives, offers ways to heal our relationships, and beckons us to return to Nature.

There is no coincidence that this book has thirteen chapters. Thirteen is a sacred number to women. The Moon makes thirteen cycles around the Earth per year. Most women have thirteen menstrual cycles per year. My intent is to present the stories and information in these thirteen chapters in a melodious, winding, weaving, encircling, all encompassing way, the way a woman thinks, the way a woman feels, the way a woman IS. Some of the chapters in this book are short and some are long, but then, this is a book that advocates change, not constancy.

"Wo-man" and "fe-male" are words used by western cultures to define the feminine gender in relation to men. We have no word in English to communicate a different vision for being female, and this lack of language reflects the existing lack of understanding of feminine principles.

Observing the similarities of our dual nature to the waxing and waning of the moon provides the most obvious description of *how* and *who* we are as females. It is the continually changing nature of the moon's reflection of the sun's light that governs the gravitational pull of the tides on earth. The continually changing nature of women governs the pull between Life and Death. Every woman's cycle contains both in perfect balance. Women are Lifegivers who intrinsically understand through the feminine principle the power and timing of Life and Death. There is no more poignant place to seek understanding of our place and our purpose on Earth. Women understand duality so well *because* we are dual. Cycles of Life and Death, guided by our own inner timing, run in our blood.

The scope of this book is to help better understand the gifts of having a dual nature and how to use those gifts to heal our relationships through dreaming, spirituality and intuition, and our innate creativity. We will look at the moist, rich, darkness of the time of bleeding, and I will re-introduce the ancient idea that menstruation is a time of purification, listening to our intuition and our dreams, birthing new ideas, and moving deeper into understanding of our own spirituality, all of which greatly enhance our relationships.

This book explores the similarities of our feminine nature to all cycles of life. Like everything in life and like the sunlight's reflection through the moon that pulls our inner waters, women are continually changing. Each change brings a gift and a different view of the world. All things in Nature move in cycles, and these cycles define Life and Death on Earth. Simple observation of Nature shows cycles in the rotation of the earth, bringing day and night, or tree rings that indicate yearly growth patterns. Scientific knowledge of cycles in all life expanded in 1729 when it was discovered that the Mimosa Pudica plant had daily cycles, closing its leaves at night and opening them in the day. Yet even as science explored cycles of life, one of the most obvious and important life cycles, that of women's bleeding, was pushed underground by the politics of our time.

We will explore in this book reasons that women's cycles have been ignored, dismissed, or pathologized, and how those actions have affected our place in society, preventing us from truly being who we are. Our Western Patriarchal society has promoted progress and constancy at the price of slower, gentler harmony with Nature. Learning to respect the wisdom of our natural cycles is a step towards healing and growth. As part of the natural universe, women have cycles that have always been with us and are the essence of life itself. It is time to awaken to the value and power inherent in another way of seeing the world, through the eyes of feminine vision.

Rather than appreciating the benefits of women's natural cycles, like ever changing dark and light of the moon, we have been encouraged to re-align our nature with a business calendar that artificially pressures us to join a linear progressive model for life, appointing nights, weekends, and holidays as the only calendar sanctioned times for rest, regeneration, and introspection. This artificial way of living has thrown our most important relationships out of balance and endangered future life through alignment with technology over Nature.

American television is full of commercials that proclaim "now you can be active every day of the month," failing to recognize the artificiality of expecting each day in a woman's monthly cycle to be the same. Not perceiving one's cyclical way of being isolates women from the processes that occur anyway; detachment from bodily changes ensures that they remain merely bodily ones, hiding unrecognized benefits.

This book will explore myths and beliefs of blood mysteries from the earliest times. The practices of indigenous peoples who are close to the land will be shared as a teaching tool;

indigenous peoples worldwide see menses as a sacred time, a time of power, where women, of their own accord, go into retreat to examine their life's purpose and to gather spiritual strength. People who live close to Nature observe that life consists of interconnected processes rather than a discrete causal relationship between things; through this understanding, indigenous peoples acknowledge and respect the natural changes of women better than their Western counterparts. In the West, the attempt to control Nature's cycles rather than recognizing that humans are part of Nature's cycles contributes to patriarchal attempts to control women through undervaluing who we are and what we have to offer.

We will explore how creativity, dreaming, intuition, and our spiritual experiences can be enhanced through deeper listening to the rhythm of our bodies and honoring their call to retreat. We will look at the benefits in each of these areas in connection to our own body calendar. Unlike the Western calendar that dictates times of rest, calendar consciousness was first developed by and in women from their natural menstrual body calendar. Chinese women established a lunar calendar 3000 years ago; Mayan women saw a relationship between the great Mayan calendar and women's cycles; in Gaelic the words for "menstruation" and "calendar" are the same. Yet with all this ancient recognition of a woman's natural cycle, modern society has chosen to try to manipulate it or ignore it.

If we are not in tune with our own rhythm, then we experience sharp and inappropriate breaks or alterations in our life's flow, expressed by many women as PMS. I suggest in this book that Pre Menstrual Syndrome is a culturally induced condition resulting from the scientific dissection of physical and emotional events that occur during menstruation and a suppression of women's emotional vision. This book combines an understanding of hormonal changes and emotional guideposts for life changes. I also introduce the idea that the power of Menopause has been squelched through lifetimes of cultural assault on women's cycles. It is through failure to listen to the wisdom of our own cycles that we approach Menopause in such confusion.

Women are central to our homes and our communities, known as lovers of peace, and the natural creators of life. When women's cycles are ignored, controlled, or denied, there are long reaching unpleasant effects. I believe that ignoring or suppressing women's natural cycles contributes to the increase of stress and illness, the deepening of sadness and depression, and greater disparity in our relationships. While each woman must evaluate the worth of these assertions herself, the evidence is clear to me. Patriarchal misconceptions have imprinted themselves into women's consciousness as truth. The smell of patriarchy is concrete, rigid and stifling, blocking us in and paving our direction. Patriarchal culture demands: cut it down and pave over it. Pour your own image into the mold and cement it into the place where Nature once cycled through the seasons.

Feminine consciousness knows to go down into dark earth and breathe in the moist stillness. Feminine smells reflect the cycles of life and death: grass, flowers, trees, ocean, stream, meadow, the fecund smell of fall leaves turning into earth; the fragrance of feminine consciousness calls us to merge with Nature. Each starting place stirs us towards the next level of birthing, the stretching forward in fullness until the core of us rips through the ground and waves our newly sprouted greenness towards the wideness of the blue, blue sky. Sweet, ripe, redness gathering into blossom, then fruit, feminine consciousness offers herself to the world to be eaten, and then drops back to earth for another cycle of being born again. We are not paved over. We do not cement our image over the ever-changing landscape, demanding to stand firm or build on the shifting sands of time. Change is our lifeblood. We need to better understand the wisdom of our own life cycles. It is time to return to the feminine and heal our relationships through living in harmony with Nature.

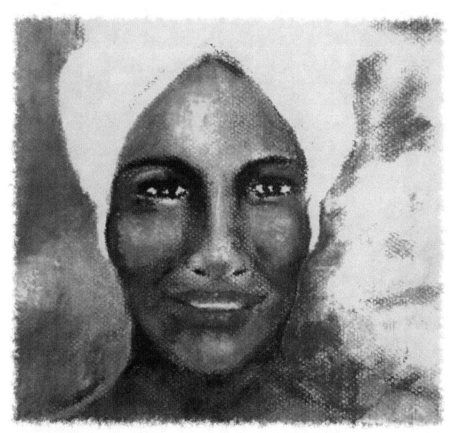

NAMING
—Rebecca Smith Orleane

I know
The shape of a word in my mouth,
Whether it sticks in my throat,
Or glides smoothly forward.
I know
The vibration produced as my thought turns to speech,
Whether words connect as they land,
Or repulse upon their arrival.
I know
The power of the words I speak,
And yes, *I* must direct
The power of Naming.

ONE:
THE POWER OF WORDS

At first glance, this chapter might appear to be all about Menstruation, but this is misleading. The underlying essence of this chapter is about addressing the dual nature of being a woman. It is because duality is dismissed as a lesser virtue than constancy, that the dual nature of women has been rejected in favor of the modern idea that *equal* means *the same as*. In disregarding half of who we are while striving to be the same all the time, we lose the creative power of being female. Naming the one natural process that is part of our biological, emotional, and spiritual nature determines whether we, as a culture and as women, accept our duality or reject it.

Before we can decide what to call something, we need to figure out what it is--and what it means to us. How DO things or events acquire their names? Generally speaking, we give events or items names according to their meaning. Each language names things according to cultural understanding or from root words that originally connected to that culture's meaning. Frequently, however, the original meaning is lost as time and speech shape the language. Some meanings are grouped together in a single word that carries related meanings for everything in the group, even though they are different. The English language does that often, causing a lot of confusion in communication. Two examples come to mind: *snow* and *love*. The Inuit language has many words to cover the varying aspects of snow (cold, wet snow; icy crystals of snow; snow with wind; etc.) There is no "catch-all" word "snow" for all the varying forms of snow and the underlying meanings of each type of condition in English. *Love* is similarly differentiated in other languages (Greek, for instance) for the varying meanings of different kinds of love. Yet in English, although the meaning is different for each, we still say we *love* our mate, our friend, our sister, our children, the place we live, and our job.

How we "call" something, it's name, announces our connection (or disconnection) to it, how we feel about it, and what meaning it has for us. Words like *snow* or *love* can become confusing because they carry so many meanings. On the other hand, some events (or things) are so big and carry so *much* meaning that we have an abundance of names to try to catch the whole meaning or to express the enormity of the concept. The concept of divinity, of a supreme being is one of these, and some of the words used to name this concept are *God, Goddess, Holy Spirit, the Divine, Great Mother, Holy Father, Creator, Great Spirit, the Infinite, and Source.*

The event of women's monthly bleeding is an event so large there are many attempts to name it. *Menstruation* is the medical term in English, but I am sure each of you can think of many other names you have heard for this event. What is it, or more specifically, what is the meaning of this event culturally and individually to us? *Menstruation.* Who does it? What does it mean?

Menstruation is a product of womanness. All women do it- teens, mothers, virgins, married women, single women, professional women, and homeless women--*all* women, regardless of race, culture, or sexual orientation. Unless there is a medical reason preventing menstruation, all women, at one time in their lives, will participate in the monthly cycle of bleeding. It begins at a certain point in a girl's life and stops at a certain point after she has experienced adult womanhood. So it is related to a particular time, and a particular way of being in the world.

Chapter Six of this book discusses the medical aspects of menstruation, offering a more complete understanding of what happens physically during this time. Chapter Two will address how the meaning of such an important event changed in our culture and how some of the more unfortunate names for such a sacred gift arrived. This chapter begins our explanation of the *meaning* held in the event of menstruation and offers some of the names that convey the meaning of the event. Naming springs forth from meaning in every culture, and through the power of naming, meaning can be changed.

The menstrual cycle is fundamentally an act of creation, of ripening, of renewal. Our attitudes and our culture's attitudes about this special time are important in our understanding and treatment of the event itself and its importance or disregard is woven into our daily attitude. Prevailing ideas surrounding menstruation in our patriarchial culture encourage discounting the monthly cycle, treating it as a time to be ignored, ashamed of, and "gotten through" as best one can or as something that is merely necessary for biological continuation. The meaning in the event is often seen as an inconvenient act of nature that interferes with human plans for what we may want to do. Born out of this dark meaning, the names our culture give menstruation are revealing of a deeper disrespect of or disconnection to Nature's gift of duality in women.

Biology has decreed that once a month women will be different than they are the rest of the month. This monthly difference marks women as being dual by nature, able to see differently and to be different according to our internal state. In a culture that values constancy, the dual nature of woman has often been denied, belittled, and even dishonored. More about that later, but for now, I want you to understand that any time something is belittled, a momentum is set in place for establishing names that reinforce the deprecation of

4

the event. Once the demeaning name is invoked, the power inherent in the gift of the event is diminished.

Over the years, I have "collected" cultural nicknames for menstruation, and regrettably discovered that almost all references to menstruation in our culture have a negative connotation. Look at the ones listed below, and see how you feel when you read them:

- the curse
- *that* time of the month
- wrong time of the month
- sick time
- monthly troubles
- old faithful
- the misery
- under the weather
- indisposed
- I fell off the roof
- the nuisance
- tide's in
- riding the Red Tide
- visitations
- Aunt Flo is visiting
- My red-haired aunt is visiting
- Lady in Red
- The Chick is a Communist (1940's jive)
- Communists in the Summer House (Norwegian)

- on the rag
- period

How many of these names have an underlying meaning that something is "wrong" with the event itself or infer sickness or injury? Probably anybody who reads this can think of even more disparaging terms for women's menstruation. Even the popular term *period* infers a stopping of something and may have negative connotations to women of a culture that values constant forward progress. Women (and girls) who experience monthly bleeding as an event perceived by society to be sick, injured, or wrong, learn to devalue the duality within themselves. They quite naturally will treat the gifts of their own duality and the event of menses itself as something to be covered up, hidden, or kept secret. It becomes an event of shame because it points to an assignation of "being different" or "something wrong". This in turn gets internalized to self-doubt and sabotages a girl's or a woman's self esteem. If something that happens through Nature relegates her to a position of being ridiculed or mocked or made fun of, she is not going to want to explore the potential gifts that come with this monthly change. This especially affects young girls whose greatest desire is "to be normal". They want to be like everybody else, and when "being normal" comes to mean not bleeding, the event is swept into secrecy and, worse, shame. Media adds to this derision of monthly bleeding through advertising that insinuates that you will be mortified if anyone discovers that you bleed (if you have a menstruation staining accident), or that you must be kept "fresh" (as if bleeding is offensive by nature), or worst of all, offering advertisements that promote sameness as if it were a virtue, such as, "now you can be the same every day of the month" (as if being different is in itself a curse.) Is it any wonder that so many women have problems with self-esteem, given that the most natural of events is referred to with such names of derision and disgust?

We need to explore more deeply the meaning of having a monthly cycle and look carefully at what names we choose to express the meaning of that event, for in denying the positive aspects of monthly bleeding, we deny half of who we are as women and the gifts we bring *through* our ability to see things differently, to be dual. Thankfully, many aware women today are re-examining the negative implications that have been assigned to menstruation and looking for the positive aspects being humans with the capacity to see things differently at different times. You are probably one of the people trying to change cultural misconceptions about this beautiful event if you are reading this book. At the very least, the book has captured your interest as a topic worthy of investigation.

From the earliest human cultures, the mystery of creation was believed to be connected to the blood women shed monthly. Noticing that women seemed to bleed in harmony with the moon, most tribal cultures in North America treated menses as a spiritual event. There was clear recognition, if not understanding, that out of bleeding, women brought forth life. Among the Kalahari Kung, a menstruating girl is believed to have great spiritual power that can be harnessed for the good of the community if rightly treated.

Assigning spiritual meaning to monthly bleeding advanced the idea that the event should be treated with respect. Indigenous women decided for themselves what would be most respectful for this time that reminded them of the moon's movement from dark to light, noticing that they, too, changed like the moon in regard to their own desires for introspection or social connection. In our earliest human history, indigenous women worldwide found that it felt appropriate to withdraw from secular duties and social connections during their time of bleeding. Recognizing that bleeding was an event that belonged exclusively to women, they separated themselves from men during the menstrual flow. As indigenous women separated themselves and withdrew from daily activities, they became more aware of the cleansing nature of bleeding and the gifts of dreams, creativity, and intuition that came from allowing a special time to become introspective during this cleansing. In short, our ancient grandmothers discovered that treating this time as a spiritual event brought special power of creation- whether the creation occurred in the birth of a child, in a beautifully woven basket, or in creative resolution to a relationship problem, it was a powerful time for bringing change.

Because of this inner knowing about bleeding and how to treat it, early indigenous women understood that they had a special power that could be used for the good of the community or could overpower and cause harm. (Chapter Four will discuss this in more detail.) Menstruating women set themselves apart from, and in many ways, above the rest of humankind. The Dine refer to the time of a young menstruating girl as the time "when she has her power." A Hopi woman elder once said, "We have power. Men have to dream to get power." It is recognizing and accepting inner duality that allows women to understand their own power. Perhaps such power was seen as a threat long ago, and the beauty of being dual was degraded. At any rate, if one sees the dual nature of women as bringing power from monthly bleeding, an entirely different meaning forms for understanding menstruation than the one our culture assigns. There are few positive names, and only a few, on the list of names to call menstruation. Notice that most of these are connected to Nature:

- Moontime
- Woman's Friend
- the flowers
- Mother Nature's Gift

My personal favorite is "Mother' Nature's Gift." For the

purpose of this book, I will shorten that label to "Nature's Gift." But first, I will speak about one of the oldest and most common references to menstruation: "moontime." Calling menstruation moontime stems from an acknowledgment that women's cycles reflect a timing similar to the moon's cycle of change. Languages around the world acknowledge the ancient relationship between women's natural rhythms and the moon's rhythms, and lunar myths provide coherent theories concerning death and resurrection, fertility and regeneration, initiation, etc. The cycles of the moon are connected symbolically to women's bleeding cycles worldwide. Native American women call menses "moontime." French peasants call menstruation "le moment de la lune;" in German country districts menstruation is referred to as "the moon;" it is spoken of as "ngonde" (moon) in the Congo; and in Torres Strats the same word means both 'moon' and 'menstrual blood'. The list of universal references to the moon-menstruation link shows that women have long understood that there is a connection to cycles of the moon and their own gift from Nature. The indigenous term "moontime," (which, or course, varies in each tribe's language) recognizes the moon's and women's times of fullness and times of withdrawing into the dark for regeneration. While some women choose to call menstruation "moontime," I discourage use of the phrase "on my moon" because they are a culturally corrupted blending of "moontime" with "on the rag".

In this book, I will refer to menstruation as *Nature's Gift* because I enjoy the feel of the words in my mouth and because the word expands upon the awareness that women shine the light of who they are in different ways during different times, honoring the inherent gifts of being connected to Nature. As we progress in exploration of women's cycles, I trust I can convey to you the positive meaning of having a monthly cycle, rather than the reigning cultural assumption that menstruation is a necessary biological inconvenience necessary for the birth of children, or worse, something to be ignored or conquered. (Patriarchal culture values conquering and controlling of Nature.) If by the end of this book I can convince you, the reader, to see menstrual blood as a magical fluid with a power to bring increased creativity, guidance, and strength, and harmony, the gates to understanding the joy and wonder of being a naturally dual creature, a woman, will be opened wide.

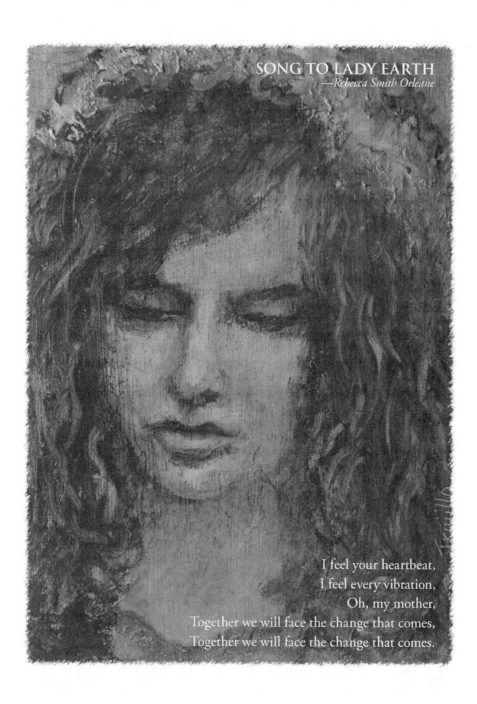

SONG TO LADY EARTH
—*Rebecca Smith Orleane*

I feel your heartbeat,
I feel every vibration,
Oh, my mother,
Together we will face the change that comes,
Together we will face the change that comes.

TWO:

RELIGION REPLACES SPIRITUALITY

When I was a ten year old steeped in the Christian doctrine of my tribe, I asked the preacher of my church a few puzzling questions. I was having trouble understanding exactly how a woman was made out of a man's rib. It didn't make sense to me that man was made first, and then woman came from a portion of the original product. Since, in my young experience, girls seemed to catch on to things quite a bit faster than boys did, and were definitely better at getting good marks in school, sometimes ran faster, and seemed more interested in making things (while boys tore them apart).... why exactly was it that we were made second? Perhaps there had been an error in the preacher's lesson that we came second "to be a companion for man." I thought perhaps really the Creator had made man first as a "practice run" and then refined the creation on the second go round.

I also did not understand why the Church was teaching me

that I should not listen to my body, that it would betray me. So far, when my tummy said I was hungry, I was. And when I stumped my toe and felt the pain, I knew to pay attention. So in what way was my body going to betray me? Little did I know that the coming menstrual cycles signaling sexual awareness threatened the Church that fed me my spiritual tenets.

Later, as I was being coached through a Southern girlhood with advice such as "Let the boy think he is smarter than you," I decided that there was something seriously flawed with that system. Why could I not just be myself? My attempts to be who I was were quickly corrected. I found there were special conventions governing cross gender interaction. To acknowledge attraction to a boy without the customary feigned and pretentious disinterest required of "the more modest sex" was paramount to spelling out that you did not know the "rules of the road" and therefore, you did not fit in—a teenage girl's worst nightmare.

It didn't get any easier when at twenty-two, and I was castigated for being "an old maid", nor at twenty-three when I finally did marry and lost my own credit records to my husband because he was "head of the house." I was outraged that I was the one working, paying all the bills, balancing the household accounts, and *my* credit record (so carefully built as a single woman) was suddenly assigned to him, a boy in school!

My questions about the order of things and, particularly,

my place as a female in the existing society, caused me nothing but trouble until I moved from the South and the politics of the times caught up to my own reckoning of the way things should work- sort of.

How did we arrive at a position of having to hide part of who we are as women? At what point did we move from accepting our nature to hiding in shame? I believe that the answers to these questions lie in the evolution of humans from hunter-gather societies to agricultural societies, and with that change, the movement from nature-based spirituality to a patriarchal religion.

In her book, <u>Rebalancing the World</u>, Carol Lee Flinders explains that hunter-gathering people upheld Values of Belonging:

- connection with the land
- empathic relationship to animals
- self-restraint
- conservatism
- deliberateness
- balance
- expressiveness
- generosity
- egalitarianism
- mutuality
- affinity for alternative modes of knowing
- playfulness

- inclusiveness
- nonviolent conflict resolution, and
- spirituality

These qualities were valued by both genders in hunter-gatherer societies. With the arrival of agriculture, they conflicted with the goals of the new patriarchal system. Rather than discarding the old values altogether, they were relegated to the domain of women. The new Values of Enterprise, as Flinders calls them, became entrenched and were passed down as the values by which we live today:

- control and ownership of land
- control and ownership of animals
- extravagance and exploitation
- rapid change
- recklessness and speed
- momentum and high risk
- secretiveness
- acquisitiveness
- hierarchy
- rationality
- businesslike sobriety
- exclusiveness
- aggressiveness and violence
- materialism

Drunk with the pleasures of ownership and control, humans began to move away from the land and their positions as Nature-beings. With the exception of indigenous cultures, which were incredulous that someone could *think* of owning our Mother Earth, our European forefathers (and mothers?) gave up the nomadic, land-based way of living and adopted a more settled lifestyle. They made a stark move away from being children of the land to being landowners. The switch from spiritual connection with the land to dominion over it bred concepts of competition and acquisitiveness. Humans, who had always shared everything with generosity as indigenous cultures do today, changed value systems with one swift discovery that being in control brought power. Under the tutelage of men, women were taught that control brought comfort, so it became more palatable, and a choice of values was made.

Being in control is addictive; it offers a strong sense of safety, and by contrast, suggests that lack of control means uncertainty. The catch here is that in the hunter-gatherer societies and indigenous cultures, uncertainty and lack of control were managed through spiritual understanding that the Earth Mother could provide for all living things and an understanding of life cycles. Everything cycled, so therefore a cycle of provision would surely follow a cycle of need.

With the coming of agriculture, indigenous beliefs and values were pushed aside or assigned to the realm of women, as humans moved from equally valuing the connection of all things to a position of dominance over the land. Mother

Earth was no longer treated as a living being supporting humans and animals and plants; to humans, She became inert land to be controlled. The first agriculturists decided which plants were "crops" and which were "weeds" and began to exert control over their placement and their growth. Rivers were dammed or diverted to control their flow. Rather than belonging to the land, the agriculturists claimed ownership and dominion over it.

The arrival of Christianity supported the rising belief that dominion was superior to belonging, and with the advent of the written word, a doctrine was born to support a new myth that man was given dominion over the land and all her creatures. With such a powerful shift from land-based spirituality to the written world of an abstract god, people lost the holiness of being a part of Nature and the importance of listening to bodily awareness. The body was caste out, as a detractor, something that interfered with the "higher" progress of humanity. This shift in lived belief was a death cry for gender equality. Women's self-esteem was dashed. Women, life givers who had enjoyed full awareness of Nature's cycles through their own bodies, lost the ability to keep the balance through their innate understanding of the creative gifts of their dual natures. On a planet where duality infuses everything, the loss of understanding of such a gift created enormous imbalance, for women have always taught by example how to honor life and death through their inner understanding of duality.

As people settled onto "their" land rather than moving in nomadic patterns, women were no longer working side by side as partners with men. The labor was divided into more gender specific roles, and men became more responsible for the decisions that were made outside the home, while women were consigned to producing sons and caring for the now permanent home.

Values of belonging are indistinguishable from worldwide indigenous values. In virtually all indigenous cultures, women enjoyed equal status with men, and in some they were even in charge. Women and the cycles of life that are part of their nature were honored in traditional indigenous cultures because women are uniquely able to bring life into the world. The new patriarchal Christian culture did its best to eliminate rhythms of life in order to instill sameness (stuck-ness, lack of creativity, death). It is worth observing that in its decree of banning birth control, even the "rhythm" method was outcast by the Roman Catholic Church. Being in rhythm with Nature became an affront to God.

In the new system, women were no longer seen as productive when they slowed down to honor their natural biological rhythms. Withdrawal from normal duties for the higher calling of bringing forth life, through pregnancy and childbirth, or through creativity of a new project or idea born from the monthly cycles that were by now seen as an embarrassment, allowed more control of external affairs by men who through new eyes now evaluated everything in terms of progress. The intuitive wisdom of women that came through their dual nature and their times of bleeding were no longer honored or respected. Their insights and ideas were no longer sought for the creativity they held; in fact, intuition quickly became something that was feared by men and hidden by women, as women were labeled witches for knowing things intuitively. Later intuition became a secondary value labeled "women's intuition", a lesser thing to be discounted in the wake of scientific evidence.

The strength required for childbearing was turned into a time of frailty. The pain of childbirth was viewed both as punishment and proof that men should not listen to women. When it was understood from the new myth that Eve had been cast from the Garden of Eden for eating from the Tree of Knowledge, beliefs were set in place to keep out any knowledge a woman might offer.

Western concepts about menstruation were influenced by patriarchal ideas exemplified by myths within the Christian church. Because Eve was taken from the rib of Adam, she could never be whole; she would always be only a shadow or a part of a whole person. In addition, the Christian church held a philosophy called "original sin" and a mythology giving Eve responsibility for the fall of man from the Garden of

Eden. This belief system has shaped the idea that women are being punished by monthly bleeding ("the curse") and pain of childbirth for tempting men to engage in the fruits of the mundane world.

As women's gifts were increasingly undervalued and discounted, even the gift of bringing children into the world became a duty to be performed for the landowner/husband. Every landowner needed sons to strengthen his legacy and continued control over larger and larger domains. Rather than nursing and caretaking each child long enough to teach it how to have an independent and connective relationship to the world, women were encouraged to produce more sons to carry the family acquisitions forward into the next generation. Slowly the power women had over producing life became another event to be controlled, and menstrual cycles became an impediment to the service of men.

As time progressed, the female values spurred political movements for equality, and the Women's Liberation Movement was born. Women gathered together to restore their place beside the men. However, in the desperate cry for equality, the pendulum swung too far in the other direction resulting in a struggle to prove that women could be more *like* men. Rather than arguing the benefit of feminine duality, women sought to prove their constancy, resulting in the imperative to hide monthly cycles of bleeding lest they be seen as inferior. Years of negative beliefs about menses fathered the view that menstruation was something debilitating, inconvenient, and undesirable, something that removed a woman from constant progress. Nature's gift was seen as biologically necessary if one wanted to a child, but otherwise it was viewed simply as an inconvenience to be ignored, a nuisance in the way of "more important" things, such as bringing home more money, building careers, or gaining political office.

The importance of women's duality and their accompanying cycles of life were almost completely lost with the advent of birth control pills. Suddenly millions of women consented to (or even asked for) the regulation of their natural cycles to be more "convenient," ignoring the appropriateness of their own rhythm. One result of this artificiality was the forcing of all women taking birth control pills to an often unnatural 28-day cycle, a severe step towards cloning with a complete disregard for individuality. With this huge shift of priorities, women lost the understanding of the importance of their own natural timing and the art of going inward when Nature called. This artificial tampering severed or badly injured women's remaining connections with their intuitive guidance. The loss of right timing and intuitive guidance, accompanied by the dismissal of women's thoughts and feelings as unimportant, lead to deeper frustration and grief for women, and Pre Menstrual Syndrome (PMS) was born.

PMS, which has become a household word in western

society, was brought forth from the cries of hundreds of thousands of Western wombs with the lack of regard for women and the superficial scheduling of sacred cycles. While there is a place in medical categories for extreme hormonal imbalance requiring outside intervention (called Pre Menstrual Syndrome), the PMS that most women believe they experience is simply the subtle announcement of moving into another way of being. The changes women undergo every month resultant from hormonal shifts occurring just prior to Nature's gift have *physical* attributes such as tender breasts, water retention, and occasional headaches. There are accompanying emotional changes in the form of increased emotional awareness. Neither of these categories of change are pathological; they are mere signals for women to slow down and honor their own cycles of life.

In my lifetime I have heard the argument that women should be disqualified from major political office (like being president) because possible PMS reactions could trigger war! It is not the physical reactions that caused this fear; it was the *emotional* changes that occur premenstrually that have hindered the assignment of women to responsible decision making positions. Luckily, that trend is changing, and women are finally achieving political posts, although not always according to their merits. Prevention of high political posts for women because of fear of emotionality is actually a tragic mistake. Emotional states are merely signposts pointing to changes that *need* to occur. (I think it much more likely that the occurrence of an emotional state during a woman's cycle or just prior would bring forth more creative efforts for peace!)

When emotions are suppressed or treated with derision, insinuations, or outright prejudicial statements, they burst out unexpectedly as the hormonal veil is lowered *because they will be heard!* Loss of intuitive guidance followed by denying emotional response is directly responsible for the origin of PMS, which outside of extreme clinical hormonal imbalances is, incidentally, a purely patriarchal phenomenon.

Further, living a lifetime of menstrual cycles without listening to emotional signs for needed change, or without consideration of the importance of a time of retreat, has brought us to the edges of chaotic menopause, where the body rebels in a fury of hot flashes and unhappy mood swings. Our hurried modern society allows no room for slowing down to allow women to naturally shed what is unneeded in their lives physically, mentally, or emotionally. If a time and space were created for women to honor the natural slowing down Nature intends, they would be better able to dream and create what is needed in their lives the way our hunter-gather ancestors did. How have women lost the understanding of this process?

At the beginning of this chapter I shared one of my early encounters with religion. Our most familiar cultural myth has shaped the treatment of women by teaching that

Eve sinned (made an error) by discovering forbidden fruits (knowledge) offered to her by the intuitive wisdom arising from the Earth Mother (the snake). Actually, the knowledge she discovered was *body* knowledge, a way to experience "heaven" through connection with another human: sex. Eve, through the tutelage of the snake, discovered how to move from duality into oneness. In other words, Eve followed her natural instincts, discovered delight of unity with man, and was condemned for knowing that she had the power to bring forth life.

To understand a culture's value system, one must not only look at the culture's behaviors, one must also examine the culture's creation myth. With the coming of agriculture, Nature-based spirituality of respect and connection could not support the emerging value system of competition and aggression. A new story was needed to uphold the new values. As hunter-gatherers began to settle into permanent communities, Mother Earth, spiritual progenitor for *all* life (and hence, female, since only females can bring forth life) was pushed aside for a new king, a divine male image that was wrathful and all knowing. Female wisdom was thrust, literally, underground. The snake, which through its ability to shed its skin had heretofore represented the ability to shed what was not needed, came to represent evil; fear of shedding, fear of snakes, and fear of women's monthly bleeding, was induced culturally.

Modern patriarchal culture fears snakes and what they represent: the abilities to shed what is irrelevant in life, to go underground for wisdom, and to bring forth new answers. Snakes and women have both been feared and dismissed in the current living myth. Since the snake has been relegated to tempter rather than wise guide in the Judeo-Christian Creation Myth, Christianity has instilled a deep phobic reaction to both snakes and menstruating women.

Because the new culture had created a myth that men were the givers of life (a male deity, a male rib forming the first woman), the idea of a woman's connection to life and death through blood also needed to be changed to support the belief that it was *men*, not women, who were important. The ancient icon of the mother pelican piercing her own breast so that her drops of blood will feed her nest of newborn chicks was usurped by Christianity and replaced by the sacrificial bleeding heart of Christ.

Sacrament is taken in the form of red wine as a symbol of the blood of Christ in the Christian church today. But red wine had been used as a symbol of the blood of the Great Mother, the Holy Woman, for centuries before Christ. In many cultures, ceremonies took place in which women and men would take the symbolic blood of life in the form of red wine-for example, in the Dionysian mysteries and Tantric rituals. Sometimes this was consciously acknowledged as being a symbol of the menstrual blood, the magical fluid out of which human life was created. Blood has always been the main symbol for the wellspring of existence and the mystery that sends us forth into this life. As such it was revered. The fact that women bled once a month meant that they were closer to this wellspring.

The shift from Spirituality to Religion required rejection of respect for women as the life givers. The newly created myth placed men in place of creator, decreeing that woman was taken from *man* as a divine event, rather than acknowledging the divinity of every birth a woman accomplishes.

Removing women from the position of divine life-givers required debasing the treatment of women's cycles as well. Part of the problem is that menstruation announces that a woman is a sexual being, and the new belief system could not support the power implied through life-affirming sexual response and sensuality. Having the power to create suggests also having the power to destroy. If woman could make things grow, she could also make them wither on the vine. Recognition of this dangerous and dual power led to disempowerment of women in the early days of the Christian church. The dogma of religion replaced the peace and harmony of Nature-based spirituality.

Perhaps we have a better understanding of how humans came to live in a way that women are viewed as less capable, more dangerous, and more delicate than men. Or perhaps this viewpoint is too scary, too threatening to look at deeply for some who are comfortable with the existing paradigm. It is my opinion that our predominant religious systems support a Creation Myth that places women in an underling position to be governed and controlled.

I look back at my ten year-old questions and sense of the world, and I understand the confusion I experienced. Of course I tried to live by the values of my tribe, and in the process I learned to deny what my body told me was true. Now, as a post-menopausal woman, I reflect on the fact that because of cultural persuasion I denied or ignored the gifts of women's cycles for a large part of my adult life. I fervently wish to prevent other women from making the mistake of detaching from or being embarrassed by their dual natures.

Personal growth is not necessarily a linear progression of increasing speed, and duality is divinely necessary in order for us to be able to see the whole from different perspectives. Slowing down, looking and listening deeply to Nature, and sharing with others frequently solve more problems and create a more harmonious lifestyle than our hurried, progress-oriented human pace. Quiet, cooperation, and intuition are values worthy of being considered and practiced. The duality of women and their accompanying cycles must be viewed not merely from a biological perspective, but from an understanding of our deep connection to the divine cycles of all life.

DUALITY AND CYCLES
—Rebecca Smith Orleane

"Which Came First,

The Chicken or the Egg?"

Never mind.

Each produces the Other

As they are intrinsically linked.

Bleeding and Not Bleeding,

Also intrinsically linked.

Each way of being makes you

You.

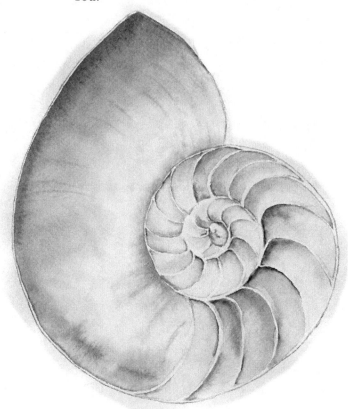

THREE:
THE CYCLIC NATURE OF LIFE

Do you remember twirling around and around and around as a young girl? I do. And I still see daughters and granddaughters doing the same joyful twirling as part of their play. I rarely see boys twirling. I think young girls are responding to the female biological imperative to move in circles as if they know that connection, or joy, or life imperative is found in spiraling around. The joyful divinity of life expresses itself in circular movement.

We move in circles through seasons and through time. Everything on Earth is interwoven into a living system of cycles. Life is a process that waxes and wanes, and does not hold up to linear expectations. Cycles of Life are systemic, and balance is maintained through these cycles. Nature, the feminine principle Herself, "refuses to be seen in absolute terms but, rather, exists in every imaginable variation" (1);

yet within these variations cyclic patterns of rhythm and repetition govern Life.

Not only is everything in life connected; there are cycles that map the most auspicious time for everything in life. Birds know when to fly south for the winter. Dolphins determine when to hunt for food and when to play according to cycles of the tide. There is a rhythm to life that makes it work. Nature's rhythm gives us the Cycles of Life. This chapter is about Nature's cycles, and I hope through understanding how *everything* in life moves in cycles, you will become more aware of and comfortable with your own cyclic nature. (Men have cycles, too, they are often just not as obvious as women's cycles!)

Almost every culture recognizes the presence of cycles representing them in circular art, calendars, and astronomy. In Greece, Pythagoras proposed a cyclical model of the heavens, and the Mayans developed a Calendar based on cycles of energy and time. Artistic representations of cyclic rhythms have been dated as far back as 4500 B.C. on Chinese vases showing self-devouring serpent designs. (The image of a coiled snake represented cyclic properties of the universe; in fact, the snake has been seen as a universal symbol of reincarnation for at least six thousand years.) Other cyclical designs have been found in Babylonia, Iran, India, and Egypt.

Ancient people believed that time was cyclic. Moving backwards in history from early Greek philosophers, who proposed a cyclical movement of the stars, one finds Biblical references to cycles. Ecclesiastes declares that there is no new thing under the sun.

"To everything there is a season, and a time for every purpose under the sun; a time to be born and a time to die; a time to plant and a time to pluck up that which is planted; a time to kill and a time to heal; a time to tear down and a time to build up. A time to weep and a time to laugh; a time to mourn and a time to dance; a time to cast away stones and a time to gather stones together; a time to embrace and a time to refrain from embracing; a time to lose and a time to seek; a time to tie up and a time to untie; a time to rend and a time to sew; a time to keep silent and a time to speak." (2)

Henry David Thoreau expressed appreciation for all of Nature's cycles advising us to,

"Live in each season as it passes; breathe the air, drink the drink, taste the fruit, and resign yourself to the influence of each. Let them be your only diet, drink and botanical medicines. Be blown by all the winds. Open your pores and bathe in all the tides of that nature, in all her steams and oceans, at all seasons." (3)

Western society today typically views time as linear, stretching from past into future, one sequential event following another. This linear view of time has had tremendous effect on Western thought, including the Western view of reality, the preoccupation with progress, views of what is "natural", and attempts to control Nature's cycles rather than recognizing that humans are *part of* Nature's cycles. Belief systems of our patriarchal culture have lead to trying to conquer the timing of cycles, focusing on history as a learning tool. Rather than accepting the inevitability of cycles in life, Western children are taught to learn from their historical mistakes and *move forward*. Learning from mistakes does not usually honor accepting the right time for action or inaction. The higher value taught by our culture is to overcome timing, following the adage "the early bird gets the worm." Never mind that the worm might be under three feet of snow and waiting until a more appropriate season might get the worm more easily.

Westerners hold a causal and linear view of reality. By contrast, indigenous cultures, model their behavior on observations made in Nature. African, East Indian, Chinese, Native American, and Aboriginal cultures all hold cyclical views of reality, believing that, like the things they see around them in Nature, reality also is cyclical. People who live close to Nature observe that life consists of interconnected processes rather than a discrete causal relationship between things. The relationship between honoring natural cycles and health and growth is clear.

As part of the natural universe, women have cycles that have always been with us and are the essence of life itself. These cycles can be a key to understanding all cycles of human nature, helping us to realize who we truly are as biological human beings. It is important to honor all natural cycles in order to deeply grasp the understanding of how non-linear Nature is.

Our human perspective of the apparent directionality of time is actually a series of cycles: the crescent moon always becomes full and then becomes crescent again. The death of one creature makes fertile ground for the birth of another. Events in Nature are not directional in a linear sense, but are circular because death and decay become the fertile ground of new life.

No one thing exists exclusively by itself; rather, all things are connected in a great cycle. Eastern, African, and Indigenous cultures recognize that life itself cycles into death and back to life again in a process called reincarnation. Time, through which these cycles can be seen, is a process, not a series of events. When time is viewed as a series of linear events causally leading towards a final conclusion, life is viewed as a series of things that happen, and the presence of cycles remains unseen.

Life is rhythmic. The rising and setting of both sun and moon cycle in a rhythm. The ocean's tides, seasons of the year, and even the stock market all function in cyclical rhymicity. Periodic behavior is especially obvious when one examines any aspect of time. More than three hundred years before the birth of Christ, Aristotle noted cyclical swelling of the ovaries of sea urchins at full moon, Hemophilus of Alexandria recorded daily cycles of pulse rate, and Cicero wrote that the flesh of oysters waxed and waned with the moon. In 1954 Eliade proclaimed that the reappearance of cyclical theories in contemporary thought was "pregnant with meaning". He stated:

"Just as the disappearance of the moon is never final, since it is necessarily followed by a new moon, the disappearance of man is not final either; in particular, even the disappearance of an entire humanity (deluge, flood, submersion of a continent, and so on) is never total for a new humanity is born from a pair of survivors. This cyclical conception of the disappearance and reappearance of humanity is also preserved in the historical cultures." (4)

Others have also asserted that since so many biological rhythms have been found, it is simpler to assume that everything is rhythmic unless proved otherwise.

To understand cycles of life, we must have an understanding of interchangeable cycles of matter and energy. Ecological cycles consist of solar energy transformed into chemical energy by photosynthesis. Each ecosystem contains cyclical exchanges of energy and resources. The cyclical nature of ecological processes is an important principal of ecology. Communities of organisms have evolved in ecosystems over billions of years, continually using and recycling the same molecules of minerals, water, and air. Quantum physics explains that matter and energy transform from one to the other and then back again in continual process. Emilie Conrad and Candace Pert assert that physical processes aren't things, but are dynamic and take place in an open, fluid system. Cycles of life are systemic, and the understanding that the living organisms cyclically flow through ecosystems is one of the basic concepts of ecology. Life is a process, not a linear series of events. Everything that happens is connected to a universal system.

Life on Earth is defined through two cyclical processes. The first can be understood as a cycle of creation and destruction, explained in life terms by photosynthesis, the building of plants and animals through the use of carbon, and their disintegration as the process continues. The second process to understand is the cycle of synthesis and degradation, where the presence of bacteria causes biological materials to cycle. Further, the natural dynamics in life can be seen in three separate circulations: nitrogen and sulfur cycles, geochemical carbon cycles, and bacterial cycles.

The carbon dioxide cycle is one cycle necessary for life to exist; volcanoes spew out huge amounts of carbon dioxide. Plants and animals recycle the carbon dioxide and oxygen through photosynthesis, keeping the atmosphere in balance for life to exist. As part of an ecological system, volcanoes, hurricanes, and other so called "destructive" forces do their work in order for life to continue on Earth.

Chaos theory shows that greater and greater complexity causes movement towards a bifurcation point, where change can occur. This point is a place of infinite possibilities that cycle around a strange attractor, called *change*. In the midst of this complexity, stable cycles suddenly return. In animals, what could appear to be randomly changing populations, are actually reproduction patterns that repeat in three or seven year cycles. Catalytic cycles are at the core of self-organizing chemical clocks of life. The lava that spews forth from the volcano becomes in time the fertile soil for plants to grow; the riverbed that overflows brings minerals to enrich the soil. From the enriched soil, life springs forth. The increased population of deer brings back the almost extinct wolves. Balance is maintained.

Like the whales, swallows, and butterflies, the lives of rocks are marked by cycles. Layers seen in rock patterns demonstrate cyclic patterns of water and rock movement. Rocks have been in motion for millions of years, shaping and reshaping the face of the earth. Plants and animals do not live apart from these movements of rocks and continents; their own lifecycles are immensely influenced by cycles of Earth movement. As the moving Pacific Plate destroys existing rocks, creating bays and deep-sea canyons, plants and animals are born, die, and turn back into rocks, cycling from plant to rock and back again, from life to death to rebirth in a different form, as their environment changes. *Movement* is implicit in Nature's cycles because motion promotes *change.* All things in Nature move in cycles, and everything is interwoven into a living system of the Earth.

Circadian rhythms (defined as inner cycles connected to the Earth's cyclic periods of day and night) abound in nature. In protozoa and algae there are 24-hour periods regulating photosynthesis, cell division, movement, and luminescence. Plants possess diurnal rhythms governing the movement of leaves and the opening and closing of flowers. Some animals (whales and swallows) migrate in a cycle consisting of a series of seasonal return migrations between feeding ranges and breeding ranges. Twice a year, the entire population of Pacific gray whales swims to and from their summer feeding grounds in the Bering Sea. Other animals (the butterfly) begin cycles that are completed through their offspring.

Humans, as part of nature, are also governed by circadian rhythms. They are important for human health, safety, performance, and productivity. The circadian clock not only regulates our 24-hour rhythms, but is also involved in the regulation of rhythms of much longer duration, such as women's monthly hormonal changes and seasonal sleep changes. Seasonal changes in night length induce parallel changes in the duration of melatonin secretion so that the human sleep cycle is longer in winter and shorter in summer. These changes in duration of nocturnal melatonin secretion, in turn, trigger seasonal changes in behavior. Behavioral changes paralleling cyclical seasonal changes can be seen in both animals and in humans.

Every part of being human includes a cycle of some sort. More than one hundred functions and structural elements in humans oscillate between maximal and minimal values once a day, including our breathe, our blood, and our hormones. It is difficult to find any aspect of being human that does not include a cycle of some sort. However, humans have done their best to ignore natural cycles, abandoning natural human rhythms for the more controlled industrial, technological rhythms of life. The technological acceleration of rhythms in day-to-day living is an affront to the human nervous system and is contributing to our separation from Nature and each other.

The age old question "which comes first, the chicken or the egg?" indicates human awareness of the presence and importance of cycles in Nature. Yet modern societies are rather determined to override these cycles, trying to control Nature rather than flowing with Her. Patriarchal societies usually think in a linear fashion, focusing on "progress," defined as moving developmentally along a line for an improvement. Every mother is proud when her child has learned to walk, indicating "progress" towards growing into adulthood. Yet this same progression ultimately leads to death, and unless death is considered as a part of the life cycle, progressive, linear thinking has a sorry end for those who are intent on conquering Nature. Death is perhaps the ultimate act of renewal! It is especially imperative for humans to recognize cyclical processes of life and death, for excessive reliance on left brain linear thought or societal structure arising from orientation towards progress alone breaks the harmony with the natural world.

Modern urban influences are changing human biological function. Related health problems are increasing as natural biological needs are ignored; when the cyclic nature of the universe is not honored, illness often results. Diseases occur as human lifestyle, diet, and medical care cycles change, and we humans pull away from Nature trying to push forward towards a sort of progress that uses us up rather than supporting our own cycles of life.

Moving away from the natural order of life seems to move the individual closer to disease. "Hurry sickness," a term coined by Julian Gresser, is the result of our restless progress away from the natural, sacred cycles of the seasons, the winds and the tides, and most directly, the rhythm of our own bodies.

In disease etiology and treatment, physicians recognize the importance of biological cycles. For example, cancer treatments take advantage of the rhythmic regulation of cell division, which contrasts with the unpredictable division of cancerous cells. Western physicians also recognize the importance of honoring some basic natural cycles in treatment such as the need for sleep and proper nutrition. However, cycles are viewed as even more important in Eastern medicine, where recurrent weather conditions such as winter cold can reactivate dormant problems, including arthritis pain, or summer heat can affect the heart. Cyclic processes are at the foundation of the theory and practice of Chinese medicine and its older sister, Ayruvedia. In the Five Element Theory, each of the elements (representing a specific organ in the body) is related to an element preceding it and one following it. Too much or too little of one element causes the next element to be out of balance as well. As each organ is affected, the one next to it is affected, completing a cycle of health or disease.

Immune, endocrine, and nervous system cycles are part of information processing for humans that make a total system. Our science is moving away from perspectives of causality and towards an understanding of cyclical systems of information. Biochemicals communicate through a non-linear process of information exchange: cycles.

Although cycles are evident throughout the universe, it is curious that one of the most obvious cycles (women's monthly bleeding) is often ignored in the West. These cycles demonstrate our deep connection to the natural world. Trying to control or suppress these cycles (as with birth control pills) or ignoring them is an act that removes us from Nature and from balance that is inherent in cycling as a part of life. We become out of balance when we argue with Mother Nature.

Like women's cycles, breathing is also a cyclical process. There is a great similarity to the design of women's cycles and breathing cycles. It is necessary to both exhale and inhale to sustain life through breathing. Likewise, it is necessary for women to experience both the letting go and the building up of blood within their bodies in order to create life. Both cyclical processes are acts of renewal. Discharging old blood and discharging used air both renew the ability to create life. Blood renews the possibility of creating life. Breath renews the energy of the body and sustains life. Both cycles are designed to alternately let out the old and then allow the new to flow in.

We can study our breath, or we can study women's cycles. Both have merit in showing the relevance of honoring the timing and versatility of Nature. I will discuss women's cycles in more depth later. Regarding breathing cycles, which are necessary for the life of all humans, not just women, it is clear to see that if one cannot breathe out strongly and thoroughly enough to allow a proper in-breath, the breathing cycle cannot function optimally: the carbon dioxide- oxygen exchange necessary for life is thwarted and life becomes a struggle from the deepest core of existence: our breath. In his excellent teaching about breathing, Robert Litman states that carbon dioxide is the master hormone of life; it regulates all activity. If we struggle to breathe, our immune systems are compromised. This understanding illustrates how deeply we are connected to the basic cycling of life within our bodies: that of carbon dioxide- oxygen exchange. When we do not fully honor that cycle by allowing ourselves to exhale (as many of us do not), we are removing ourselves from being fully functioning biological human beings. We become mechanized because we are not connected.

Automated human beings are literally "not running on all cylinders." They lack depth and cannot relate to others because they are disconnected from their own nature. Look at yourself and notice how you breathe. Notice how others around you are breathing. How many of us caught in the urgency of continually pushing ourselves forward to the next task, are really able to breathe? If we listen closely, can we hear the spaces where we are holding our breath, waiting for something or afraid that we will not meet the demands society places on us and we place on ourselves. Can we notice how often we take breathe in but don't exhale? The lack of honoring of cycles and the linear focus of living in a progressive society enhances the tendency to grasp at everything and hold on to it, even our breath. We don't really know how to let go of what we need to release in order to allow space for the next thing, the next breathe, to come. The fact that women in modern cultures try to push through days when they are bleeding and releasing as if they were ordinary days shows how severe is the problem of being unable to let down, to breathe out, to rest.

Our relations with others also reflect whether we have balance or not. All people interact with others, whether it is through intimate partnership, children, family, neighbors, work, or relating with strangers. In relationships, attachment and separation are part of the cycle of human life. It is easy to see cycles in infancy and childhood, as children gain increasingly broader discoveries about themselves and the world. Each new realization brings a child back to the place of new questions. Cycles are also easy to see in adolescence, as the search for the balance between identity and intimacy appears; teenagers can be seen moving into and out of each repeatedly.

Adult cyclical interactions are not always as obvious, for in our society, relationships have been romanticized by media to the point that partnerships often times become "throw-aways" the minute the fairy tale stops, rather than working through the cycles of highs and lows that intimate relationships offer as a way of growth. Often, the minute the relationship dips out of "being in love" to the low places that offer the opportunity to grow through looking at our own fears and shadows, the relationship is thrown away rather than honoring the cycle of change.

As people change and different situations occur, partners weave in and out of love and work. A set of partners may work different jobs, handle different chores, or have different hobbies, all separate and individually, only to come together in love and intimacy as they share their day or discuss their children. A good relationship is a process of continual change as it reflects new issues, deals with challenges that arise, and uses the resources available at each stage of life. Most humans cycle in and out of needs to be alone and needs for companionship. Healthy relationships recognize that cycles occur as part of the relationship, like everything else in Nature, and honor the importance of each stage of the cycle.

There are cycles that map the most auspicious time for everything in life. Women are fortunate enough to have an internal map that gives them directions on the most promising times for everything they do. Unfortunately, our western culture has decided that women's inner guidance system is obsolete, and has re-programmed women to follow the timing of a modern prescribed calendar, a calendar operating seven days a week, as opposed to following the timing of our own bodies in accordance with the timing of Nature.

It often may seem inconvenient to follow Mother Nature's directions. Many women wonder how they will get everything done if they stop. But if we don't allow the exhale, the rest, the movement to the downward part of the cycle and insist on keeping a consistent, forward moving pace, we find ourselves exhausted and we are robbed of the energy necessary for our creativity. We have been persuaded and allowed ourselves to believe that to keep up with all that we wish to accomplish, we must follow a calendar dictated by men. Our current belief seems to dictate that in order to survive in a man's world, women must not only adopt a linear-based masculine calendar, but also insist that their bodies conform to a 5-day-on, 2-day-off artificial cycle. Because women are continually encouraged to be the same and advised that inconsistency is a detriment (just look at any feminine hygiene advertisement on TV or in a women's magazine), we have devalued our own inner rhythms.

The portion of a woman's cycle that pulls us more into ourselves in order to cleanse what we do not need and to change what is not working is usually viewed as a time of general disgruntlement, where women's perceptions are identified as problematic. Emotions that come more easily during the inward part of the cycle are discounted as being part of PMS, rather than being valued for what they might actually be saying about a woman's life.

While Premenstrual Syndrome (PMS) is a clinical medical diagnosis, our culture has adopted the policy of assigning *all* cyclical changes in women to "PMS", ascribing culturally negative values to inherent positive attributes. Television and magazine ads promote constancy with slogans like "Now you can be the same any day of the week." I'll have more to say about that later. For now, just remember this: when women strive to be constant rather than honoring their own cycles, their full potential is diminished.

Ignoring a woman's cyclical nature isolates her from processes that occur anyway, knowledge of which may very well bring balance and benefits. Detachment from bodily changes can lead to repression of the benefits of those changes. With loss of connection to one of Nature's most powerful rhythms, women may lose the sense of balance within themselves, their relationships, and their world.

Women grow through cycles in the same way that the moon grows through changes and cycles. The moon rules the flow of fluids (both ocean tides and individual body fluids), including the timing of the menstrual cycle, the fertility cycle, and birthing labor. Cycles specific to women offer an opportunity to truly understand the magnificence of being part of the natural world and enjoying differences that bring special gifts. The nature of women is cyclic; we are dual creatures who have the natural opportunity to understand life from both external movement in the world and inward movement within ourselves.

Women's fertility (which can be defined as any type of creativity) waxes and wanes each month. As creatures of duality, waxing and waning cyclical processes guide us. If we are not in tune with our own rhythm, then we experience sharp and inappropriate breaks or alterations, rather than as a cyclical steady unfolding.

I accept that the universe is cyclical in nature, and therefore, looking at everything in it in a cyclical fashion rather than linearly gives me a clearer view of what might be true. I also know that understanding the importance of women's cycles in relationship to the cyclic universe is critical. Women, known as lovers of peace and the natural creators of life, are central to our homes and our communities. We can no longer allow the essence of who we are to be hidden under the patriarcial rug.

If we ignore, control, or deny the importance of our own cycles and our dual nature, there will likely be long reaching unpleasant effects. I believe we are seeing some of those unpleasant repercussions today. It is very possible that ignoring or suppressing our natural cycles is contributing to our increase of stress, a lack of connection within relationships, the greater frequency of illness, the deepening of sadness and rise of clinical depression, and a decrease of creativity on all levels (including infertility and intuition). While each woman must evaluate the worth of these assertions herself, the obvious connection of women's cycles to cycles of all life must be acknowledged. Through a feminine understanding of all cycles, all of us (women and men) can learn a great deal about how to live with respect for each other and for all of life; we *are* part of Nature.

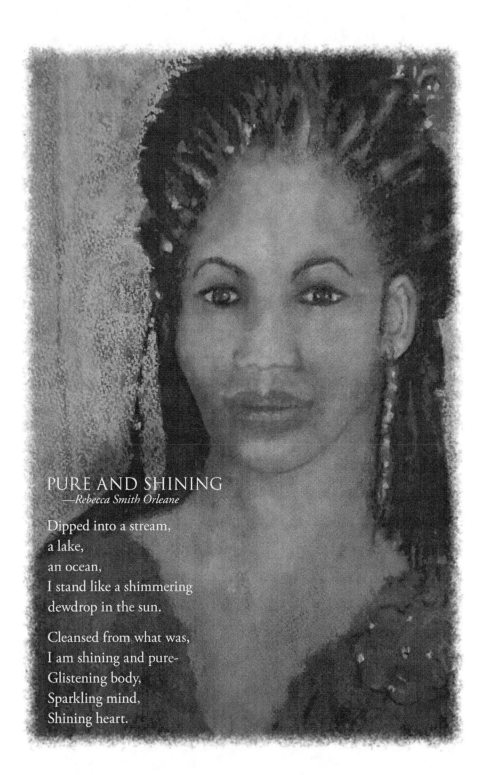

PURE AND SHINING
—Rebecca Smith Orleane

Dipped into a stream,
a lake,
an ocean,
I stand like a shimmering
dewdrop in the sun.

Cleansed from what was,
I am shining and pure-
Glistening body,
Sparkling mind,
Shining heart.

FOUR:
BLOOD MYSTERIES

I was standing in the Stanford University Park, staring at the enormous statues carved by the men of Papua New Guinea. Huge penises and men with wombs. Penises with a bowl beneath them and carved figures of gods emerging. I was standing in the midst of a living creation myth, stories pouring out of the art like the blood they depicted. In Papua New Guinea, it is believed that while women can give birth to children through their blood, men give birth to the gods through male blood. Since men do not have a monthly bleeding cycle, the male kings ritually slit the underside of their penis and drip blood into a bowl, ceremonially giving birth to the gods. They see this act as the secret of creation, for without this ritual, the gods would not be born and so, the world would no longer exist. Starring at the statues, I was in awe at the depiction of the jealous longing of the men, a longing so strong it produced imitation of women's monthly bleeding by the men, particularly by the king.

Throughout history, blood has been seen as an important connection to life and to death. Whether blood is produced through wounding or flows naturally, as in menstruation, every culture in the world gives meaning to the flow of blood. Most people have strong beliefs about blood, beliefs that have been passed along through stories, which may be the same for women and men, or which may differ. Each civilization passes down these stories, or myths, about life and death, about blood, and about the balance of power between men and women. Because the meaning of blood differs from culture to culture, treatment of men's and women's blood may also vary from culture to culture. Islamic peoples think of all blood as something not quite whole. Chinese people say that blood is polluting because it flows out of the body as a waste fluid. Indigenous people from all over the world see blood as carrying the power for change, and modern Westerners are confused about blood; many Westerners seem to be captivated by the presence of blood (as evidenced in the abundance of horror movies) or they are indifferent and removed from its meaning. Whatever the cultural position, blood stands for life, so the shedding of blood can be frightening, dangerous, or mysterious. I will share with you some cultural and historical perspectives about blood, menstruation, and the balance of power between women and men. It's an interesting tale, no matter what its cultural spin.

We'll start by looking at male and female views of menstruation; next we will investigate a few myths about blood and power; we will end this chapter with a deeper understanding of the balance between life and death.

WOMEN'S AND MEN'S VIEWS OF BLOOD

Women and men have different views of blood. Typically, men think of blood as being connected to injury or death, a symbol of something being wrong. Women, in modern culture, have been taught to also view blood as an indication of something gone awry, and thus, they often feel inferior whenever they bleed themselves, as if their act of bleeding is a statement of something being amiss. It is a fairly recent state of affairs for women to believe they are wounded, hurt, or inferior whenever they discharge lifeblood. In fact, if you ask most modern Western women to address their view of blood, they will speak of blood with revulsion, as in blood produced from injury, violence, or war, or as a nuisance, as in the blood of their own monthly cycles. Often it seems they would like to ignore blood or wish it away. While the aversion to blood from injury or death has not changed much historically, modern views about menstrual blood are very different from the view of our ancient sisters!

In most cultures women's menstrual blood is considered to be very different from blood that comes from injury or death, although the connection is clearly apparent: from blood new life springs forth; shedding blood indicates death, whether it is a child that is not to be, or actual death resulting from wounding. Women have a special perception about the meaning and cost of shedding blood; we understand at a bodily level the vulnerability of human flesh. How easily it can bleed! The natural processes of menstruation, childbirth, and menopause initiate us into deep understanding, perhaps in a way that a man can never conceive (pun intended.)

In most indigenous cultures women are aware of the effect of the gravitational pull of the moon on them and their blood. Women *feel* fuller and emptier at certain times of the month. Gravitational pulls of the moon also have an internal pull; like the moon, women can feel the tides in their own bodies, whether they heed this rhythm or not. Because women's bodies (which are three-fourths liquid) routinely release and replenish their blood, they notice the pull of the moon more than a man would, like creatures swimming in the ocean feel the ocean tides more than does land-based life.

Men's views of blood throughout history have been linked to power. Men in traditional roles have been warriors and hunters who have seen the loss of blood as a step towards death, and usually, they were the ones to initiate the bleeding. Male views of menstruation, accordingly, reflect loss of blood as a step away from life. Islamic men consider menstruation as a wound. According to the Qur'an, even though menstruation is natural, it upsets people's sense of what is whole. This view of women's bleeding also elicits a tender concern for women. Hurt, vulnerable, women can elicit from men an instinct to take are of them. In Islamic cultures, the importance of women's blood is seen in the cultural requirement that a non-elastic hymen be present and capable of producing blood upon first sexual penetration. The importance of the hymen's capacity to bleed profusely makes it the most essential part of a girl's body. In Islamic culture women's blood is somehow connected to honor.

In Egyptian culture blood is also connected with honor. A new husband pays the bride's mother for maintaining her daughter's honor with thirty Rials in cash and the bloodstained handkerchief he produces after the wedding night. Punishment for lack of blood on the wedding night is harsh and can lead to the girl's being killed by her family in the name of honor and virginity. Doctors do not often get a chance to see different types of hymens, since gynecological examination of virgins is rare. Therefore they are liable to make costly mistakes. Clearly this gap in understanding the female body is costing some of our sisters dearly, even today.

Male misunderstanding of women's bleeding has been problematic throughout history. Male beliefs about menstruation have varied culturally through time, yet it is generally agreed that men have traditionally viewed menstrual blood with awe or fear. The fact that women could produce blood monthly and not be wounded caused reverence in some cultures and fear in others. In those cultures that feared menses, menstrual blood was considered to have power. The Gimi of Papua New Guinea saw menstruation as a constant threat to male purity and superiority because menstruating women are so powerful. While some tribal men believed blood *could* be powerful enough to bring death, most North American tribal men approached menses in a spiritual way, as a power that could bring good *or* evil. Men made room for Nature's gift in their lifestyles for the sake of their women, family, and nation. Many African tribal men also used this approach to menstruation. A "Master of the Earth" of the Beng in Africa said,

> "Menstrual blood is special because it carries in it a living being. It works like a tree. Before bearing fruit, a tree must first bear flowers. Menstrual blood is like the flower: it must emerge before the fruit- the baby- can be born. Childbirth is like a tree finally bearing its fruit, which the woman then gathers." (5)

A spiritual approach to women's bleeding honors and allows women to have a greater sense of their own power.

Anthropologists writing about menstruation have argued that the sight or thought of a person who bleeds from the genitals (a menstruating woman) could be frightening to a man, who naturally protects his protruding genitals, and through, as part of his protection ideology, has an intense castration anxiety. Others have embraced the view that men were generally frightened by any loss of blood and reacted by trying to avoid it. Yet while avoiding blood, men were envious of women's capacity to bleed from the genitals without being wounded, and blood initiation rituals to emulate women's blood-making and child bearing powers were born from this envy. Many modern day men view menstruation with a mix of awe, fear, and/or revulsion. As I have previously stated, the Judeo-Christian religion has fostered a view of women as unclean, lesser beings. Today orthodox Jews refuse to shake hands with a woman because she might be menstruating. According to the Laws of Manu, if a man even approaches a menstruating woman he will lose his wisdom, energy, sight, strength, and vitality (a clear recognition of women's power reflected through fear-based beliefs.) Traditional Chinese have a similar reaction to menstruating women, since they think of all bodily discharges as unclean, dirty. Menstrual blood in Chinese culture while seen as powerful, is viewed as particularly unsanitary, because it is directly connected with human procreation.

Whatever past or present male beliefs about menstruation, reasons supporting those beliefs have been lost in many modern societies. Respect and reverence for the ability of women to bleed without injury as a natural phenomena has been replaced with analytical examination of chemical changes or ignorance and confusion surrounding this most precious of times. Many men today are left wondering just exactly what women's monthly cycles are all about.

BLOOD AND POWER

Since flowing of blood always brings change, time has born the understanding that blood holds the power for change. Most, if not all, ancient societies came to believe that blood held power, particularly menstrual blood. The blood of menstruation has been referred to as sacred or supernatural throughout many ancient cultures. The idea that a woman could bleed regularly without having been wounded and without dying scared men. In Europe and in colonial America, women's menstrual power was so feared by men, that a myth of witches was created, producing a legacy of harming women rather than honoring them. Women's innate connection to Nature and the intuitional wisdom that came from their deep listening frightened the men who wished to be in control. Not long after the inception of the myth that wise women were witches, puritan beliefs born of a patriarchal doctrine prohibited discussion of menstruation or other bodily functions; the holy power inherent in the changes brought by women came to be feared rather than respected. The community fires that women had knowingly avoided during their bleeding cycles were used to destroy powerful women, as they were cast into the role of witches.

Reaching further back into history, we find that when understanding dawned that women were able to create new human life through blood power, Mayan men, like the New Guinea men, thought they could create the birth of gods through offering their blood. The king was believed to have the most potent blood among humans; therefore, he was the focus of tremendous power. A gift of his blood was thought to bring the gods to life and divine power into the lives of the Maya.

In most ancient cultures the power of blood was neither bad nor good, but merely dangerous because of the change it brought. It was not *necessarily* harmful, but it *could* be harmful if not treated properly. Indigenous people knew that because blood holds the power of change, that change could go in either direction. In fact, the Cherokee believe menstruation is *symbolic* of change, and change can be either good or bad. Therefore, during Nature's gift, women isolate themselves so that their power will not affect their community. Menstrual blood, according to Cherokee tradition, is a child that has not been born. Therefore, menstrual blood intrinsically holds the power to bring about change. Cherokee women take measures to seclude themselves during menstruation and childbirth because both events involve blood and are considered to be associated with a spiritual power that is so strong it can overwhelm medicine, spoil crops, or incapacitate warriors. Before reentering society, they neutralize themselves with water. Their voluntary seclusion is one way they signify their power. Consequently, men respect the danger and keep their distance. Only the women know about the rites they perform to control and channel their own power. In Australian Aboriginal understanding, menstrual blood is sacred and powerful. Here, too, men avoid menstruating women so they will not be overpowered by this potent, holy fluid specific to women.

Other cultures believe that the power of a menstruating woman may cause anything to change, and women who have not learned to channel this potent energy have little control over their power. In Portugal a menstruating woman is avoided because it is believed that her powers for change could cause plants to wilt or objects to move inexplicably. Menstruating women who have little or no control over their special powers can bring chaos to their physical environment simply by their presence. Celtic myth holds the belief that a drop of any falling blood, whether male or female, is dangerous and has corrosive powers, causing infirmity. The ancient Celts believed that only if it were mixed with heart could its corrosive powers be neutralized. The Kalahari Kung of Africa believe that a menstruating girl has great supernatural powers that can be harnessed for the good of the community if rightly treated. Believing that the power of blood is able to provide for their needs, they use the blood of a menstruating girl to bring luck to their men when they hunt.

All blood is seen as powerful in Chinese culture because it is a life-giving substance. Menstrual blood is triply potent; it has inherent power; it is necessary for the creation of life; and it has the power to cleanse when it is discharged as waste fluid. Because a menstruating woman is temporarily the bearer of a powerful and potentially harmful substance, Chinese men and women see the presence of menstrual blood as disturbing to the gods.

Beliefs about the power of blood have led to specific treatment of blood and bleeding women. (You may explore this in more depth in the appendices I have added at the end of this book.) Generally ancient cultures honored menses as a sacred time, a time when women, of their own accord, went into retreat to clear negative energies, gather spiritual strength, and seek creative life situations. Supporting the time of isolation and relief from chores is an act of respect.

Historically, many Native American societies considered a menstruating woman to be both sacred and dangerous. Yurok women secluded themselves during the flow because it was believed that a woman was at the height of her powers during Nature's gift. The Dine (Navajo) also referred to menstruation as a time when women have their power. Around the age of ten Dine girls were prepared for the power they will possess. They were taught by elder women how to avoid harming others. The Dine believed dangers from menstrual blood increased with age. By contrast, the Anaishnabe believed menstrual blood was more powerful in a woman's first cycle. According to them, first blood held so much power that it was possible for plants to die if touched by a woman shedding this powerful blood or fish to die if she entered a lake or stream. Because she was considered so powerful and could unintentionally cause harm through her power during Nature's gift, an Anaishnabic woman would not even look at anyone except female elders, for her glance could cause unintentional direction of her power. Lakota women also took protective precautions by isolating themselves and not interacting with the rest of the family during menstruation. Paula Gunde Allen summarized,

> "Women who are at the peak of their fecundity are believed to possess power that throws male power totally out of kilter. They emit such force that, in their presence, any male-owned or -dominated ritual or sacred object cannot do its usual task." (6)

Menstruating women were considered to be in the midst of their own powerful ceremony, a ceremony of life, so they avoided other ceremonies during menses. A Hopi woman elder speaking of men's and women's power said,

> "We have power. Men have to dream to get power from the spirits and they think of everything they can-songs and speeches and marching around, hoping that the spirits will notice them and give them some power. But we have power....children. Can any warrior make a

child, no matter how brave and wonderful he is? Don't you see that without us, there would be no men? Why should we envy the men? We made the men." (7)

The power of menstrual blood has often been misunderstood in Western culture, which filters its view through Christian myths about childbearing and sin. Contrary to Judeo/Christian beliefs, menstruating women are not polluting or unspiritual, but rather they are so powerful that they could change the shape of the world. When a woman's menstrual blood is flowing, this blood is full of the mysterious powers that are related to childbearing. To bring a child into this world is the most powerful thing in creation. A man's power is nothing compared to this. Men need to respect that power, because at this time, women *are* particularly powerful. During Nature's gift women should have a special place where they can get a rest from regular chores out of respect for this great mystery. Women have this special power because they are the only ones who can bring life into this world. It is the most sacred and powerful of all mysteries.

LIFE OR DEATH? SEEKING BALANCE

From the Pueblo Indian sixteenth century view, the world was made by throwing a clot of blood into space, thereby bringing power into the earth. The Dine (Navajo) believe first menstruation is a symbol of the restoration of power and fertility on earth and a cause for great rejoicing. The Acoma Indians believe that plant and human seeds alike hold the potential to generate life. Seeds planted in Mother Earth or a child planted in its mother's womb repeats the cycle of life. In all indigenous people there was and is a clear recognition of the need for balance, both between life and death, and between genders.

The necessity for balancing the power between men and women is reflected in indigenous cultures worldwide. Only in patriarchal societies do women struggle to maintain their own power so that the balance between genders is equitable. In Native American societies, women may segregate themselves on certain occasions, but on other occasions men are also segregated. Every ritual depends on a balance of power. It is understood in indigenous cultures that a woman's power and a man's power are opposites like hot and cold or day and night. Men's power is typically more related to fire and women's to water. Water can quench a fire, and during Nature's gift a woman's water is particularly cold. Both genders understand the principle behind ritual separations: that fire and water do not mix.

The other aspect of seeking balance with blood is the connection between death and life. From the earliest human cultures, the mysterious magic of creation was thought to reside in the blood women gave forth in cycles of Nature. Maori myth says that human souls are made of menstrual blood. Africans myths speak of the congealing of menstrual blood to make humans. South American Indians believed all men were made of "moon blood". The Aboriginals accepted salt water as a substitute for the mother's regenerative blood since it came from the womb of the sea and had the taste of blood. Superstitious fear of spilling salt was directly related to the idea of spilling blood. Pliny called menstrual blood "the material substance of generation." (8)

Aboriginal people believe that death and initiation are the same thing. The blood of birth is inseparable from the blood of death or the blood of menstruation. Because of the difficulty of separating them, all three occasions of bloodshed are considered dangerous, and the need for balancing the power between them is paramount.

Blood-Power; Life-Death; Balance. All these important concepts have been shaped and woven by our myths. Rituals support our myths, and lack of rituals construe a lack of meaning to important events. I doubt if many women reading this book had a special ceremony for their first menstrual cycle. I doubt if many men had sisters who had special ceremonies. Perhaps a handful had someone tell them that now they had a special place in society and that they should be honored whenever they were experiencing Nature's gift. The idea of honoring our cyclical nature is foreign in our culture. Most of us are (or have been) embarrassed, at best, if our cycles were noticed.

There can be no doubt that blood is related to power, and as such it should be respected. Shedding blood monthly, from the indigenous perspective, gives women the power to renew themselves. Such understanding of the connection between blood and power has been present from early aboriginal beginnings. Worldwide, women elders have taught young menstruants to seclude themselves, not because they are dirty, as Western culture has often said, but because *such a powerful time should not be wasted* in mundane tasks and social distractions. A menstruating woman's energies would be best applied as a time for the accumulation of spiritual energy, for women are the keepers of spiritual understandings about life and death. Yet our culture suffers from an embarrassing lack of respect for this holy time. Blood rituals teach understanding of and honor for change, and life is nothing if not full of change.

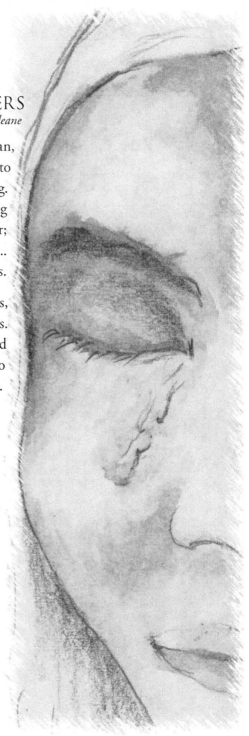

RHYTHMIC WATERS
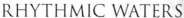
—Rebecca Smith Orleane

Salt tears, like Ocean,
Coming forth in waves to
The Beach of our Knowing.
Misty, soft, hints of Something
Deeper;
Sobs of Deep Longing...
Or Loss.

Waters of Awareness,
Pouring from our Inner Wells.
Watering our own Land
So that we may grow newly into
Who We Are.

FIVE:

CLEARING AND CLEANSING

A man once told me that a bidet is very good for women's health. I felt anger creeping up on me, flushing my face and stirring my emotions beyond discomfort. It took me days to completely understand why I was feeling angry about such a benign statement that was said so respectfully in a good conversation.

The first thing that I realized about my distress was that I felt a flash back on a lifetime of being told I was dirty. If a man were telling me my vaginal health would benefit from being washed off by a modern day appliance, then perhaps I was being told once again that I *needed* to be washed. I reacted to what I heard because my ears were full of being told I was unclean. The truth is that we were merely talking about cleanliness for men *and* women, but I took it personally. Personally for myself and personally for all women. We are not dirty.

The second understanding came to me days after our conversation. I was standing in the shower (many of my epiphanies come in connection to water) and I suddenly knew. I was mad because a man might have known something about my own very female body that I did not know myself. I was mad because I have spent a lifetime hiding from what my female body told me about what she wanted or needed because I did not want to defend her. *My* body. I grew up having to hide menstruation because it was considered dirty, and I did not want to think of myself as dirty. In my youth, if the topic of menstruation came up, it was fair game to deride a girl as a lesser being, ruled by things that made women weak and impure. Girls couldn't do certain things when they were menstruating, so girls were considered undependable. Boys were always dependable. Girl's sensitivities were greater during menstruation, so we were considered imbalanced and weak. Boys were strong and constant. In short order, girls were *less than*.

Later, sexuality was also disallowed. Not OK for girls. I grew up hearing "boys will be boys" and "a man's gotta do what a man's gotta do," references to the undeniable sexual imperative men were allowed to not only own, but to experience with no responsibility. Women, on the other hand, were raised with the Christian mythology that sex was only for procreation, to be saved for and contained within the sanctity of a church blessed marriage. The act of sex was to be experienced in "missionary position," the position of service to the man and service to God, and the only blessed way to experience sex. Women were, after all, the ones who caused the downfall of men. Our direct connection to Earth and our direct bodily awareness of connection to the divine through our sexuality was squashed with tales of the woes of childbirth that were visited upon us because (we were told) we had sinfully led men astray. Actually, we were leading men *towards* God, not away from God, or Source.

I think that even women's multi-orgasmic ability was threatening to men, who were done with their sexual need after their semen was released. The pleasure men experience has an end point. The pleasure women are capable of experiencing continues with no start or middle or end. It is a timeless association to a divine state of being, a way of experiencing oneness with another human and oneness with God, or Source, at the same time.

There is a Pink Floyd song that reflects the cultural classification of sexuality with women as dirty. The song says, "I need a dirty woman. Oh, I need a dirty girl." The implications are that the man needs sexual release, and a "nice girl" (as we were called in the South) would not have sexual desires.

The biggest sin in the Garden of Eden myth was to take away the wisdom and understanding women offered to men and to condemn it as wrong. Because from the male point of view, women are able to experience something more, it is scary business. The man is not totally in charge. The best way to end that fear was to tell women that sex was not for pleasure, but for procreation. Women were cast from the mythical Garden of Eden by condemning their ability to have and bring pleasure and by denying the wisdom they gained through their understanding.

I have since considered the modern sensibilities of having a bidet. I realize that because a man brought the idea into my consciousness, I do not have to reject it. And the suggestion is not associated to the Southern Christian mythology in which I was raised. I came to realize through that experience how deeply our belief systems are impacted by what we have been told and what we have experienced. It is our responsibility to examine our reactions when something triggers a response, such as my conversation about a bidet did. We must *know*, not believe, that our bodies are clean and pure and that we know best how to take care of them ourselves so that we are not threatened by old patterns of belief about who we are as women. We must eliminate old ways of thinking about ourselves in order to claim the fullness of who we truly are. I am thankful to the man who brought me that one time brief conversation, both for allowing the cleansing of yet another place Christian culture had polluted and for suggesting something that I may yet consider as a benefit of modern life.

The day I realized the depth of stigma I was carrying about being a woman who bled every month, I started looking more deeply at the cultural assumptions that still lived in my body. First of all, I did not recognize that having a monthly cycle was a natural event that connected me to all of life. Secondly, I was still suffering under the misconception that as a daughter of Eve, I was less deserving than men, and that I needed to *compete* with men in order to *prove* that I was "good enough."

Women have been so wounded by allowing a dysfunctional myth to create their reality that many of us struggle in a place between proving that men are wrong or dismissing male viewpoints altogether. And it is not only men who have caused the deepening of these wounds. Women have passed the hurtful misconceptions from grandmother to mother to daughter through the generations. In our most loving female relationships, we have attempted to protect our daughters by teaching them the ways of the world *as we understood it,* rather than showing them who they really are as manifestation of divine feminine nature.

The most damning part of the myth in my opinion is that women are dirty: dirty in our sexual desires, dirty in the menstruous stuff we shed monthly, dirty in our unpredictable emotions. There is a whole list of associations that spring forth from feeling or being treated as though we are dirty. The first association promotes inequality, for if we are dirty, how can we be around others without contaminating them? Being dirty automatically implies a lesser status. How can we be equal and bring gifts of wisdom if our wisdom is tarnished by the belief that we are dirty? This unspoken misconception has been passed down through the religion of our fathers. The myth claims that Eve sinned and contaminated Adam by her dirty little action. A new myth needs to be born from the greater truth: Eve claimed the wisdom of her divinity and offered it to Adam in order for them both to experience the unity of Source. The snake, which has been misaligned for offering the mythical apple of knowledge to Eve, is actually a representation of the body based wisdom and sensuality arising from a connection to Nature. We should revere snakes, not fear them!

The most important association to the current Christian myth is that if we are impure and lesser than, how can we be sacred? How can we be true to our divine nature? Right away, we can see the problem with respecting ourselves and demanding respect from others. Women's desire to be treated equally has been skewed, leading to a victim mentality of envying what men can do rather than appreciating our own unique abilities and accomplishments.

A simple and rather silly example can be seen in how women dress in men's pants (rather than feminine skirts), supposedly for comfort, and then complain because it is easier for men to urinate than for us. Men can stand up to urinate and we cannot. While it is true that male bathroom lines move more quickly than women's, the understanding of why we squat has been lost. We have lost the understanding that the squatting position is a biological advantage for women, enhancing the strengthening of muscles required for childbirth. There is a spiritual component to the way we were designed to urinate as well. Spiritually, we bend closer to Earth to blend our water with the waters of Mother Earth. But respect for our differences has been lost in the struggle to be like men. We could (and I have often promoted this idea) shorten our own bathroom lines by wearing skirts with no underwear (gasp, horrors!), thereby allowing the vagina healthy breathing rather than constricting our vessel in tight pants that have no air circulation. We could teach our daughters the truth about squatting: that it tones and strengthens our thighs, hips, and bellies. And bathroom lines? Any woman could hike her skirt and squat as quickly as a man can unzip. Equal does not have to be same!

Moving back to the more central topic of this chapter, it seems that most Western women believe that their feminine secretions are problematic. As proof of our believing *on some level* that our discharges and we are dirty, we have bought the Madison Avenue propaganda that we must cover our own natural smells with artificial douches, lotions, and perfumes. We have listened as the television and women's magazines have labeled secretions as embarrassing, and so, we feel embarrassed. If we believed our own smells were clean and delightful, why would there be such a huge market for artificial products to sweeten our scent? The repulsion of our own scent is so extreme that many women are not comfortable without using perfume as part of the their daily costume *every* day. It is hard to find a woman's product of any kind that is not perfumed. Lotions, hairspray, dish soap, and douches, all are perfumed. Our culture delivers a strong message that we are not clean enough the way we are, and we must do everything possible to cover our scent.

We have dismissed the importance of scent in navigating our lives. Although recent research has pointed out that pheromones are responsible for our (like all other animals) attraction to or repulsion from the proper mate, we have dealt with this new information by creating chemical scents that we consider better than our own. We use these scents both to mask who we are as dictated by our smell, and to attract another, any other, for chemical scents do not distinguish us. Artificial scents cannot be aimed at attracting the right match; they effuse themselves around us regardless of how our natural body might be reacting. The obvious outcome of such behavior is to choose a mate (at least on the level of smell) according to artificial standards because we have blocked our own pheromone guides. Is it any wonder that so many marriages fall apart or partners lose interest? There is no biological glue to hold the couple together after the initial sexual heat has worn off. Additionally, society praises a man who sweats, as if male sweat is proof of a productive lifestyle, or a job well done. A woman who sweats, however, is frowned upon, for our fairy book ideology says that we are supposed to smell like flowers all day long. And so, we adorn ourselves with chemical scents to represent a cleaner, fresher, sweeter version of ourselves.

The Christian Bible states that cleanliness is next to godliness, and missionaries have been scrubbing away natural scents to sterilize any possibility of our finding divinity through natural pheromone interaction. We have on our own added the excessively sweet artificial scents to our too finely scrubbed clean skin. And so, women today have arrived at a sorry point of missing the holiness of their own smells, sterilizing and cleansing away anything that might reflect upon them as being dirty. This applies to the scent of menstruation as well as the pheromones produced mid-cycle when we are seeking hormonal coupling. In indigenous cultures, scent was recognized as valuable for guiding men and women to the appropriate time of coming together or keeping apart. It was not because women were considered dirty; in fact, the scent of menstruation has been welcomed as a symbol of fecundity in earth-based cultures. It is only in our sanitized Western culture that we have adopted the viewpoint that all of our natural scents must be obliterated.

When I was almost through my years of having bleeding cycles, someone suggested to me that there might be a benefit of sleeping separately during menstruation. I learned that worldwide, indigenous women had instituted this custom for themselves and generally felt that the cycle of Nature's gift was a time of power. In addition, these earth-based women generally *chose* not to be around men or other non-menstruating women during Nature's gift. They stopped all daily tasks such as cooking and child care to go to a lodge to meditate, make crafts, dream, or commune with other women who were bleeding. Men were excluded. This time was understood by women and men alike to be a special time of purification, *not* of something dirty, but purification *from things no longer needed.*

Once I heard that menstruation was considered a time of purification, I spun back towards the vestiges of my Christian youth where I was taught that *my* blood was dirty. My immediate reaction, as you can imagine, was that I was once again being told that my body's discharges were dirty. Nevertheless, I decided to try it; when my next cycle arrived, I abandoned my usual routine and moved into a separate space to meditate and dream while I was bleeding.

Initially, the separation from others and from routine was a difficult adjustment for me. With nothing from my daily routine to do, I had ample time to come face to face with all the hurtful ideology I had been carrying for most of my life. My Southern Christian upbringing had taught me that it was not polite to mention the word "pregnant", much less to speak about monthly blood. If you were carrying a child, you were "in a family way." If you were having Nature's gift, you were "under the weather." I don't think the South is the only part of the country where menstruation is or has been considered something too private to discuss, something that causes boys to giggle and girls to be confined from certain activities because they are considered "sick." However, I received my education about being a woman in the South.

The age of thirteen not only ushered in the angst of being a teen-ager, it also showed me that now I would experience the pain my church promised as a curse for being female. My body was racked with violent cramps every month; I could never predict when I might be embarrassed by turning my clothes bright red with the sudden onset of monthly bleeding. Dirty jokes and comments about being a woman were proliferate among teen-age boys. The general opinion seemed to be that once a girl started her period she was considered both "dirty" during menses and fair game for sexual pursuit the rest of the time, a confusing message for a young woman. I became one of millions of girls who desperately needed to hide whether or not we were menstruating.

So when in my later menstruating years I heard about ritual separation, I decided to try it. As I sat alone with my own thoughts for the successive days and nights each month, I was flooded with painful memories, associations, and assumptions about who I was as a woman. I found that all that time alone once a month, rather than being a respite from the cares of daily living, gave way to unpleasant thoughts and ideas about menstruation that had accumulated from the years of my upbringing. Each month, all the old issues surrounding being dirty, different, or sexual came coursing out of my consciousness along with my monthly bloodshed, as I secluded myself in my private space. I remained perplexed at hearing Nature's gift referred to as "purification," and I battled with what I thought was an underlying assumption that I was dirty. The monthly event I had been negating all my life was full force in my face, after I had (I thought) successfully swept it under the carpet of denial. I faced the shadows of my own thoughts about menstruation.

As I persevered through the months of my experiment, I experienced huge sweeps of emotion. Some months I managed to maintain an attitude of feeling special, and I stayed in my sacred space the entire time of Nature's gift. Other months I bore the weight of feeling dirty, and I crept back into the family space in a welt of tears, feeling abject failure. On those nights, the cultural stigma of a good Christian upbringing clung to the very fibers of my being, and I could not shake off Eve's shame.

I had an additional impediment to my perceptions about menstruation, for I had never born a child. Since the Church had instilled in me the belief that my value was defined by my ability to produce progeny, the absence crushed my very tenuous self worth. And so I bled, month after month, crying over what could not be, feeling the unfairness of the cramps that would not yield a child.

I believe that a woman who bears children inherently has a more direct understanding of the importance of bleeding. No matter what society or religion might tell her, she can hold the life she created in her arms and know the truth. However, that deep, inner knowing can be, and frequently is, bent by the cultural assertions that override what one carries inside once the magical moments of mother-infant bonding have passed. Motherhood often becomes a constant giving of oneself at the expense of recognizing one's own value, and Nature's gift once again becomes an inconvenient impediment to what needs to be done, or a moment of relief at not being pregnant.

After months of trying to understand my own cycles, I had a very meaningful dream during one of the nights of Nature's gift separation. In my dream, I was told who I *really* was and of what I was capable. On that night I no longer felt ostracized, or lonely, or dirty, or anything except proud to be a woman and connected to all that is. On that night I learned that women have a power to connect to guidance through dreaming. On that night I learned that it is necessary to move old things out of the way in order to make room for the new. Finally, I understood that menstruation is the precursor to creation, and that I could recreate myself every month, letting go of everything that held me back from being my full divine self. This, I understood, was the real purpose of menstruation! This explained Nature's gift as a time of purification; it is an *opportunity* to release what is not needed and no longer works in our lives on a regular basis so that we may creatively bring forth what is needed next. Once a month women have the opportunity to rid ourselves of what is unwanted or unneeded, not just the blood, but all the emotions and hurts and conflicts that have accumulated from the last month. At last it all made sense to me. What emerged for me in ensuing months of my chosen separation during Nature's gift was a better understanding of my own cycles, my feminine spirituality, and the appropriateness of right timing in everything. I embarked upon a five-year study that turned into the dissertation for my Ph.D.

For five years I read voraciously everything I could find on menstruation, especially pieces written about indigenous understanding of menstruation. However, indigenous people don't write about sacred things, so much of what I found in print was viewed through the eyes of anthropologists, who were usually men! I broadened my approach by visiting and speaking with indigenous women who are living today to find the answers I was seeking. What I found both enlightened me, and it made me sad.

I traveled through the northern hemisphere, reaching through time to find the elders who held the mystical teachings about Nature's gift, offering myself as a woman who wanted to teach women's wisdom to the starving Western women who are in need of such teachings to bring them back into balance. I met with Cherokee, Blackfoot, Cree, Crow, Navajo, Ute, Pueblo, and Swinomish native women. I spoke through interpreters to very old women who only knew their own language. I visited women in gatherings where men were forbidden to go. I spoke with African and other indigenous women visiting America from their own countries. Everywhere I went, I entered deep conversations with women.

One of my favorite times of sharing occurred with a Blackfoot woman in Canada. It was summer, and the drive across Canada was beginning to feel long and hot. I decided to stop at the Head Smashed In Buffalo Jump Museum, a place that despite its name, tastefully and reverently told of a way of life among the Blackfoot people. As the name suggests, the museum was situated on top of a hill where long ago Blackfoot hunters had herded buffalo over a cliff. After the buffalos were killed by the fall (or as the Blackfoot believe, the buffalo offered themselves for the people), every part of the buffalo remains was prepared to sustain the tribe through the coming year. At the parking lot for the museum, a steep ascent below, a shuttle bus picked up visitors and dropped them off at the museum.

I parked my car and waited on the bus, which arrived shortly. I climbed in offering a warm greeting to the woman driver. The woman driving, nodded to me, and started driving. As we began the drive up the hill, I noticed that I was the only passenger. The driver approached the museum, passed it, and took a sharp turn leading out of the park. I sat curiously waiting to see where I was being taken, but I said nothing, respectfully waiting for the journey to unfold.

Silence filled the air, punctuated by pops and rattles as the bus made its way out into the countryside. We traveled for about twenty minutes in silence. Oddly, I was completely at peace about this spontaneous journey and cheerfully open to what was going to happen next. The woman driver turned off and headed towards a hill I could see in the distance. Finally she turned to me and said, "Spirits told me to take you to our vision quest site. This is where our young men go to quest for a dream, to get life guidance, a ritual quest that brings them into manhood. We are stopping in the distance because it is a man's place. You have questions about women. What would you like to know?"

At the invitation, I eagerly told her that I was researching women's menstrual customs so that I could re-awaken the ancient tradition off treating Nature's gift as a sacred time. I told her I felt that modern cultures had lost the sacred meaning of Nature's gift, and I wanted to help women find it again. I asked her to share whatever she wanted to about menstrual customs of Blackfoot women.

We entered into a very deep conversation where she shared with me her tribe's understanding of menstruation, the taboos established by the women, the rituals taught and practiced by the women, and stories of men's respect for the power that menstruation brought to the women. She graciously explained that Nature's gift was the same as a vision quest for men: a time of seeking, a time of listening to the spirits. She told me that if you listened, you could get answers not only for your own life, but also for the whole tribe. Nature's gift was considered a holy ritual where women separated themselves in order to better hear what was needed, both in their own lives and in the lives of others for whom they prayed.

My newfound friend explained to me how important it is for women to honor the monthly timing of listening, so that problems don't get too big or go on for too long. She told me that it is our job as women to keep things in balance, and if we are out of balance ourselves, we cannot keep balance in the community. She explained that we are the keepers of relationship, and if we don't listen to the spirits, then we don't know what needs to be done or how. Both Blackfoot men and women know this and respect the wisdom that the spirits offer to the women during Nature's gift, their sacred time of power. When women come back from their monthly menstrual vision quest, it is honored just like a man's coming back from his vision quest. The people want to know what she was told.

As a Blackfoot woman matures and learns better how to listen every month, the wisdom comes through more and more, and she learns what and how to share what she has been given through listening during Nature's gift with the community. The menstrual retreat accomplishes many things: clearing the woman of the old, opening her to listen to spiritual guidance, and seeding her with creative ideas for the future. The spiritual connection is very important not only for the woman, but for everyone with whom she comes in contact.

My Blackfoot teacher told me that women used to share a place to bleed together, away from the community, but in modern times, each woman had to find her own way to listen. The lodges of old no longer exist. She did not tell me what happened to them, but I think I know. I thanked my friend, and we began our journey back to the museum where we parted company. It was a moment of female bonding I will never forget. I cannot remember what I saw in the museum that day, but I will always remember the vision quest sight and the shared conversation with a Blackfoot sister.

What made me sad about my discoveries was how much of the mystical understanding of menstruation and the gifts it brought to women has been lost. I spoke to a young Crow woman who spoke fluid English but did not understand that Nature's gift was anything other than something that happened once a month to have a baby. She shook her head when I asked about rituals or teachings about the topic, and told me that in her culture, those things had long been lost. There was no one left alive who knew the secrets or the meanings traditionally passed down by the grandmothers.

I found other tribes where the Christian influence had forced women's rituals underground. At a women's gathering on an unnamed Pueblo in New Mexico, I found the women hesitant to answer my questions, for fear of being discovered by the men. In hushed whispers, they shared that women were only allowed to gather to make crafts, and that any hint of talk about women's matters today caused punishment by the men. Two grandmothers unhappily shared with me that women's lodges had been forbidden since the Christian missionaries had arrived over three hundred years ago. They told me that today, men were the only ones allowed to gather for ritual, and that the occurrence of any women's rituals was cause for being beaten (something unheard of in ancient indigenous culture). They were eager to share what they remembered, while simultaneously imploring me not to let anyone know where I got the information.

Cherokee and Cree women have survived the loss of women's rituals, however. While the traditional moon lodge has been lost, the understanding of the importance of separation and honoring a time of cleansing and purification has not been lost. Women of both tribes quietly remove themselves from daily activities, and allow the special time of menstruation to bring forth its gifts. The Cherokees recognize that change (which monthly bleeding certainly brings) can be for better or for worse, and they regard any potential change with some apprehension. Cherokee women therefore attempt to control its direction through separation and women's rituals. Modern understanding matches historical information:

> "Because they were the embodiment of fertility, women occupied a particularly precarious position in Cherokee society. They were dangerous because they were powerful: that is, they were capable of bringing about change in the family and in the community through the addition of a new, unknown member." (9)

Through self-imposed seclusion, women attempt to control the danger of bleeding and to minimize its negative effects. War, hunting, childbirth, and menstruation all require strict rules of behavior for the Cherokee because they all involve blood. The Cherokee view of blood stems from their belief that it contains life. If unleashed, the spiritual power that blood contains can be dangerous. Historically blood helped define the Cherokee as men and women, through menstruation and childbirth, hunting and warfare. These definitions through blood still exist, and therefore Nature's gift still retains respect. The polarities of woman and man are considered to be so opposite during a woman's cycle, that women do not risk contact with the men.

Menstrual blood, which represents fertility, is associated with cold. Therefore the cold of a woman's menstrual period is incompatible with the heat of fire. Menstrual blood is considered stronger than the fire; thus it can nullify the heat of the fire, thereby extinguishing it. Additionally, one would not want to combine the energy of discharge with the energy of creation, so during Nature's gift a woman would always separate herself from creating food or the fire that cooks it.

Traditional indigenous women have always understood the importance of honoring the opportunity that arrives once a month for cleaning out what is no longer needed. Traditional men have watched as women withdraw to take a personal inventory, cleanse emotionally and physically, and emerge with a bright new countenance and creative ideas. Because indigenous men could see the benefit of this process, yet did not have a biological opportunity for such a powerful cleanse, they created special ceremonies such as the sweat lodge for the purpose of their own prayer, meditation and cleansing. They wanted, like the women, to be able to release what was not needed and open the space for creative guidance. The Plains Indian Sweat Lodge and the Cherokee Plunge, once the purification rituals of men, today function to serve both genders as a place of routine clearing and prayer.

My own adventure into ritual retreat during Nature's gift to allow natural physical and emotional cleansing surprised me by dispelling the old beliefs I had held. The taboos previously assigned by the Christian church out of fear that menstrual blood was harmful or dirty had aligned me with most women of my time desperately trying to hide the biological fact that we were ever different. Through my interaction with indigenous women and through my own experience, I learned about the gifts a monthly natural cleanse can bring. What I learned had nothing to do with being dirty, to my surprise! I learned that retreating to a separate space during menstruation was an idea conceived of *by* women *for* women as a way of honoring the opportunity go inward and cast off whatever was unneeded emotionally or mentally while simultaneously shedding old, unneeded monthly blood.

Women have been given a natural time for cyclical purification that occurs every month. Interestingly, before electric lights and birth control pills skewed our hormones, women cycled with the moon every month, going into the retreat of Nature's gift during the dark of the moon and sharing with the community during the light of the moon's fullness. In the dark of the moon women shed the monthly linings of their wombs when babies were not formed, cleaning up and making the way for a new baby to form during the next cycle. With the sweep of unused blood, out streamed the flow of unneeded emotions. Women were able to cry over what was wrong in their lives, sleep in the dark listening to the whispers of their dreams telling them what was needed, and emerge to create new ways of being that were more fulfilling for themselves, their families, and their communities.

I hold Western culture accountable for the uncertainty and unhappiness I felt throughout most of my life about being a female who has a monthly cycle. Nowhere did I hear any encouragement or see any example of women who were proud of their natural cycles. The closest example I had for being proud of being a woman was from the women's movement that stated women could do anything a man could do- and better. That may be true, but it wasn't the point. Hiding from who we are and from our connection to the earth, to the sun, the moon, to the ocean, to all things of nature that cycle is unnatural.

Modern attitudes surrounding menstruation held by both American boys and girls are negative. Menstruation is seen as disgusting or a nuisance, or as something that increases emotionality and physical discomfort. A large percentage of girls hold on to menstrual taboos of not swimming during menstruation or not discussing menstrual issues with males with no idea of why these taboos might be appropriate. There is no modern day ritual to honor a young menstruant, to tell her that this is when she should develop sacred power, that the swimming taboo might be the only thing that is left of ancient beliefs that a young menstruant should not look at water because she is so strong that her power might change the water.

Today we have forgotten all the reasons for having a monthly cycle. Bleeding is often viewed as an inconvenience, interference in life that weakens women from the real reason for being. Actually bleeding is an opportunity to cleanse, to purify, to make a new place for creation, whether that creation be a life, the greatest of all miracles, or whether that creation be a new idea that will bring more harmony into daily living. If we don't clean out the old, unwanted, toxic, and unneeded, we have no room to grow something new, to create something better. The cleansing of our bodies (both physical and emotional) is absolutely necessary to creation on any level. You don't cook a magnificent meal when the kitchen is still littered with the dirty dishes from yesterday's creation.

Purification. It is a holy word. It means eliminating what is not needed, allowing ourselves to become so "sparkling clean" that we have a new slate upon which to write. All is forgiven, in both ourselves and in others. We have a chance to begin again- a new cycle.

And about forgiveness. Having the opportunity to forgive and start over does not mean that women must accept something that is unacceptable. It means that instead of using all your energy in anger over unfairness or inequity, you use the strength you have gained through purification to effect change, to compassionately explain why something is not working or is objectionable, or if conversation does not elicit change, to walk away from the situation and begin again. Purification is to expel what is intolerable, both in your own behaviors and in relationship to others. Purification and forgiveness are bedmates. If you practice one, the other follows.

The most powerful benefit of purification during Nature's gift today would be to rid the cultural pollution surrounding this most magical time. To purge all skewed religious and cultural beliefs that cause women to be ashamed of the duality of their being, to purge all the Western misconceptions harbored by girls and women alike today, would surely be a divine blessing. As I close this chapter, I want to suggest that each girl or woman reading about purification examine the ideas that may be polluting your own self-esteem as a woman. Do you need to withdraw into seclusion and purify your mental and emotional self to make room for the real you? And I encourage each man who may have been drawn to read this book to encourage and support the return of awareness that women, like men, are truly divine.

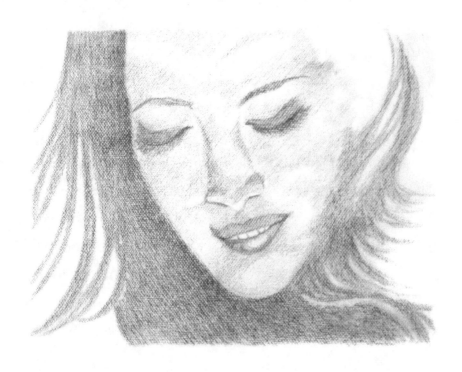

HER BODY KNOWS
—*Rebecca Smith Orleane*

A woman's body knows
What,
When,
Where,
Why,
How.
Yes. A woman's body knows.
If her body's wisdom is heard,
There will be peace in the home.

SIX:

BIOLOGY AND MEDICINE

If we delve into the understanding that cycles are the fabric of Nature, looking in depth at the biology of women's cycles can increase our wisdom about how to live as participants with Nature. The currency of Western patriarchal culture is progress, and progress assumes continual advancement. Retreat, the opposite of advancement, is considered failure. By this standard, women, who have a natural biological urge to retreat, are encouraged to be always the same in daily living. To be reliable, it seems, has been inundated with a necessity for constancy.

American television and women's magazines are full of commercials that proclaim "now you can be active every day of the month," failing to recognize the artificiality of expecting each day in a woman's monthly cycle to be the same. Failure to perceive one's cyclical structure isolates women from the processes that will occur anyway, knowledge of which brings balance and benefits. Detachment from bodily changes ensures that they remain *merely* bodily ones, while harmony with them could lead to increased wisdom about of one's nature and one's place in Nature.

Almost universally there is acknowledgment of a strong link between the moon's influence on the earth and on the natural cycles of women. The symbolism and connection of the moon to women's cycles is apparent. Environmental cues such as light, the moon, and the tides play a role in regulating women's menstrual cycles and fertility. A majority of women begin their menstrual periods during the dark of the moon, beginning to bleed between 4:00 a.m. and 6:00 a.m. Like the moon, women go through a period of darkness each month. Yet while we accept the inevitability of phases of the moon, natural phases experienced by women are not accepted for their many benefits.

To understand the differences experienced by women throughout the phase-cycle (which relate to and help us understand cycles of *all* humans), we must understand how hormones operate within the human body. Webster's Dictionary defines a hormone as a product of a living cell that circulates in body fluids and produces a specific effect on the activity of cells remote from its point of origin. Ford defines hormones as "chemical messengers, sent out by the endocrine glands, which control or stimulate hundreds of vital processes and act on almost every cell in the body" (10) Vliet refers to hormones as "chemical communicators" that carry messages to and from all organs of the body. (11) The menstrual cycle presents a picture of the constantly changing hormonal environment. Sichel and Driscoll define the menstrual cycle as "the result of an intricate, precise dialogue between brain and ovaries." (12)

Hormones influence our growth and development, mental alertness, and sleep patterns. They affect every aspect of our being, from gender to personality. Hormone receptors are more prevalent in certain areas of the body, including the limbic area of the brain (which controls emotions), the breasts, and the uterus. These hormone receptors transmit information into cells' DNA, allowing important chemical changes. When hormone levels are low, their receptors decline in number. The estrogen receptors increase and decrease depending on the phase of the menstrual cycle.

The menstrual cycle occurs approximately every twenty eight days, on the average, with day one being the first day of flow. Medically, women's cycles can be divided into the luteal phase, from ovulation until the onset of menstruation, and the follicular phase, between menses and ovulation. The first part of the menstrual cycle up to ovulation is called the follicular phase. During this phase, growth and development of an egg occur biologically; the prepared egg is propelled into the fallopian tube. Progesterone is almost absent at this time. During this time the endometrial lining in the uterus gradually builds up, preparing to receive and nourish the egg in the event that pregnancy occurs.

Just before mid-cycle, estrogen levels drop precipitously, and luteinizing hormone (LH) is released in a mid-cycle surge that causes ovulation. Ovulation brings an abrupt rise in the neuropeptides of follicle stimulating hormone (FSH) and luteinizing hormone (LH). If physical conception does not occur, the uterus lining is expelled in menstruation, and the cycle continues into the luteal phase again.

More than forty recent scientific studies show the magnitude of changes during the menstrual cycle, including temperature and hormonal changes, dream cycles, behavior changes, and mood differences. A woman's temperature cycles diurnally; it is consistently lower at night than day, and seasonally is lower in October and November than in May. This pattern appears regardless of ambient external temperatures. Women prefer higher room temperature during the luteal phase of the menstrual cycle than during the follicular phase, and in the morning as compared to the evening. Additionally, there are both quantitative and qualitative differences in the circadian levels of peripheral blood immune cells during different stages of a woman's cycle.

Tryptophane metabolites are elevated during both the luteal and pre-menstrual phases compared to the follicular phase of women's cycles. L-tryptophane is a precursor of serotonin. It is quite likely that the interaction of gonadal hormones with the serotonergic systems contributes significantly to behavior and mood changes during the menstrual cycle. Such strong biological markers indicate, to me, a very real and necessary change in women's ways of seeing the world.

There are numerous studies showing that women perform at a higher level in tests of articulation, mental arithmetic, manual speed skills such as finger tapping, and simple repetitive tasks during the follicular phase of their cycles. Plasma estrogen levels are also elevated at the ovulatory phase. Furthermore, specific aspects of memory may also covary with plasma sex steroid levels across the menstrual cycle. My own studies found a statistically significant increase in creativity during the follicular phase of women who allowed themselves secluded, quiet, introspective time during the menstrual phase of the cycle.

Additionally, women show differences in their dreams according to their monthly cycles, with increased REM periods, a greater requirement for sleep, and a sense of feeling better if they sleep longer during the premenstrual phases of their menstrual cycles. Likewise, sexual content of dreams changes with hormonal changes of the menstrual cycle. In my doctoral research, I found a statistically significant increase in the number and meaning of dreams in women who secluded themselves in a sacred space during menstruation. There appears to be a relationship between the level of estrogen in a woman's body and her degree of dreaming, as well as her memory of her dreams.

Many hormones cycle through the human body (female *and* male) on a daily level, following circadian rhythms. Additionally, it is a biological fact that many hormones act as neurotransmitters in humans, particularly FSH and LH in women. Both women and men produce the hormone testosterone. Testosterone levels cycle daily; these levels are highest in the morning, on awakening, and fall by as much as one-third to one-half throughout the day. Testosterone levels also rise and fall with experiences of success and failure. It may surprise some to find out that sexual experience stimulates a rise in testosterone more for women than for men.

Other hormones, estrogen and progesterone affect nerve cell functions. Thus, it makes sense that they would have profound influences in behavior, mood, and the processing of sensory information during the menstrual cycle. Understanding that hormones influence how we interact in the world, both as women and as men, could be profoundly important in our accepting our place as part of Nature. Women have a biological opportunity to help men understand the importance of hormonal differences for all of us. As already explained, during the menstrual cycle estrogen builds up in the lining of the uterus, and progesterone breaks it down when pregnancy doesn't take place. Estrogen produces progesterone receptors and primes them to work; progesterone can switch the estrogen receptors either on or off. These events are constantly happening, back and forth, on and off, giving women the opportunity to experience varying ways of being in the world from a biological, hormonal viewpoint.

Many women indicate that they feel more positive mood states in the follicular and ovulatory phases than they do in the luteal and menstrual phases of their cycles. The luteal phase, from ovulation until the onset of menstruation, is the time women are most in tune with what isn't working in their lives. By denying the importance of this period of different perception, women remove themselves from Nature's link. Once they have removed themselves, they no longer have assessability to their own power as teachers, for the knowledge they contain within their bodies, the knowledge of the connection to life and death, is the most potent wisdom women can offer. Once we deny what we know intrinsically, we disempower ourselves from our role as teachers, and we allow the world to continue on a path that sickens us to the core.

Are we supposed to be Stepford women, who are always pleasant and smiling? Or are we supposed to honor the darker mood states that govern our understanding of what is wrong in our homes or in the world, in order to encourage much needed change? I am not willing to adopt the medical viewpoint that women should simply accept a diagnosis of hormonal imbalance for all the dark places we may reach emotionally on a monthly basis. Quite possibly, we go along our usual paths accomplishing what we will for half the month, and then we stop, go inward, look at our lives, and assess the changes that need to occur. If we as a gender do not take this path consciously, then unconsciously our tears and anger erupt and are labeled as pathological. We are completely remiss if we simply accept the label and mask our symptoms, rather than acting on them. Perhaps the world that is struggling and so far out of balance has greater need for our dark sides, our tears of angst, now more than ever before.

The study of women's cycles has been big business in recent years. While offering great insights into the science of how our bodies work, the traditional medical model of looking at women's cycles has driven us even more towards living from a position that there is something wrong with our nature that needs to be corrected, controlled, or medicated in order to be healthy and whole. Thankfully, alternative wise women doctors like Christiane Northrup argue against the male dominator model of medicine. We have taken birth *control* pills to regulate when we bleed. Common word usage defines the thinning of the veil that brings tears for what needs to change as a "syndrome."

The lack of attunement to the monthly cycle in combination with the milieu of patriarchal need to control Nature, causes artificial hormone suppression and hormone surges, rather that the natural ebb and flow. This "jolt" in making what should be a natural change every cycle shocks women into overactive states, which our culture calls PMS.

What should be a time of sensitivity and increased intuition for a woman in tune with the cycling of her own body can become a well of sadness and misdirected anger. The attempt to control when we bleed (or how much), the desire to follow culture's direction to treat every day the same rather than honoring differences (systemic homogenation), the total disregard and lack of understanding of the reasons for gift of menstruation has caused us to devalue, dislike, or ignore one of Nature's most beautiful and valuable gifts.

While Premenstrual Syndrome was originally defined as a hormonal imbalance occurring infrequently in women, and only in severe conditions, where a woman's hormones were clinically irregular, common usage of the term has led women to believe that PMS is a natural part of being female. Monthly differences that occur as a *natural* difference are now commonly viewed as pathological. The Diagnostic and Statistical Manual (which I like to call the Pathological Bible) lists Premenstrual Syndrome as an imbalance in the hormonal system of women, consisting of specific symptoms of depressed mood, tense or anxious mood, frequent tearfulness, persistent irritability or anger, decreased interest in usual activities that may be associated with withdrawal from social relationships, difficulty concentrating, feeling fatigued, marked changes in appetite, insomnia, breast tenderness, headaches, bloating, and a sense of being "out of control". These "symptoms" occur in a cyclic pattern, beginning before menses and ceasing abruptly once bleeding has begun. The traditional medical community has accepted the diagnosis, and unfortunately, many women now believe that any of these symptoms are treatable offenses.

Traditional medical practioners have been slow to follow the lead of alternative champions, like Dr. Christiane Northrup. Instead, women's natural hormonal shifts have been pathologized into a diagnosis of hormonal disorder. Western society views women as victims of their hormones, blaming every difficulty that arises during the premenstrual and menstrual phase on hormonal shifts, rather than recognizing that the presence of hormonal shifts could allow clearer vision of what needs to change in women's lives. Rather than using emotional responses as cues to turn inward and examine the challenges in their lives, many modern day women accept the label "PMS" as a convenient way to dismiss the truth of their feelings and the necessity to bring changes into their lives.

Premenstrual Syndrome is a phenomenon that does not exist in indigenous cultures. Earth based cultures understand and appreciate the fact that when a woman is in the process of cleaning out what no longer works (uterine lining along with problems of the past month), the veil between everyday understandings and guided understandings from being in an altered space are very close. It is extremely unfortunate that such a delicate connection has been so maligned and labeled a syndrome, and that the accompanying emotions are dismissed as only an outward sign of a hormonal shift. Tears of a woman during Nature's gift are much more closely related to the salt tide of the ocean; they have the possibility of washing over us with the profound effect of pointing out that something needs attention in order to change. Female emotions during bleeding have no business being compartmentalized and relegated to the back room of science as "mere hormonal changes."

There are a number of studies that report a significant cyclical difference in the level of mental distress women experience. Is it any wonder that mental distress is so present when the dictum of normalcy does not allow a woman to be sad or angry? Of course we feel mental distress if our feelings that something is wrong are not validated, if we are continually told that our unhappiness or discontent are medical problems. All we need to do, we are counseled, is wait it out because it is "only" PMS or we can take a happy pill and make it go away. There is absolutely no place for accepting unhappiness as part of the cycle that promotes change in our culture. This philosophy applies to men as well, many of whom are medicated with mood elevating drugs rather than examining what is not working in their own lives.

How can ignoring such prodigious differences in any way honor the naturalness of who we are, either as women or men? The very appearance of women's menstrual bleeding and its temporary stoppage during pregnancy indicate a powerful influence over life. Men have cycles as well, for the muscle content of men is largely made of water and all of our brains are primarily made of water; both muscle and brain are susceptible to the gravitational pulls of changing tides of our planet. As far as I am aware, there is little or no research about the emotional cycles that occur in men in resonance with the phases of the moon or other governors of Nature; however there is much documented information about cyclical changes in women, who naturally exhibit dual nature through our monthly biological changes. We desperately need to understand the emotional changes that occur in both genders as pointers to necessary change, rather than pathologizing them as Depression or PMS. Cyclical emotional releases (whether they are connected to women's monthly cycles or men's undetected cycles of emotion) are signposts pointing the way to change if we open our eyes and look at them.

If depression is only treated with pharmaceuticals rather than examining its underlying causes, it can only take one further away from living an authentic life as her true self. If attempts are made to artificially control menstruation, pathological problems frequently manifest. Traditional Western doctors routinely give young women oral contraceptives creating artificial cycles (birth control pills induce bleeding every twenty eight days when a woman's natural cycle may be every thirty or thirty one days), rather than recommending contraceptives that do not interfere with the cycles of their own bodies. Oral contraceptives have been shown to eliminate part of women's hormonal communication pathway, including the sexual communication with men. Women on the pill do not secret the volatile fatty acids in vaginal secretions (known as copulins) that stimulate male sexual interest and behavior.

Why are there so many misunderstood aspects of menstrual cycles, in spite of clear biological evidence? Most scientific studies indicate differences in women at various times in their cycles, yet some studies cannot pin down the difference, calling it "self-reported," and others deny a difference conclusively. Obviously, the very linear Western scientific approach to studying women's cycles is not the best approach for understanding natural cyclical processes. Modern society needs a more holistic view of both women and men, as part of a more holistic view of all of Nature. If women's cycles are taken apart and studied in pieces, by hormones or behavior or mood differences, there will always be a lack of total understanding of those natural cycles. Linear designed studies will always draw conflicting conclusions because of the failure to see the whole picture. In order to elicit accurate understanding, the entire process must be taken into consideration. Biological and psychological processes must be appraised in conjunction with the woman's view of her natural cycle and the viewpoints surrounding her from her family and community.

Understanding women's cycles has the potential to offer universal understanding of cycles throughout Nature. How we relate to women as they change can teach us more respect for Nature in all her forms as She changes. It is so obvious when looking at the seasons of the year that Nature decrees a right time for everything. As humans, we may participate in that timing; we may pick berries in the summer and read by the fire in the snowy winter. Yet we fail to participate in the natural timing of our own cycles, preferring instead to separate non-popular aspects of femininity and label them as something to correct, something to bring in line with more pleasing aspects of being feminine.

Much of the fear-preventing acceptance of women's natural cycles is related to a larger fear: death. Death in any form is only part of Nature's cycles. The fact that women know so clearly that death is intimately connected to life causes great discomfort in our culture. We are able to accept that leaves fall from trees, decay, and new leaves come again in the spring. Yet death connected through blood appalls us, and we turn away from women's blood as if it will contaminate us with the scent of death by its very presence. Death comes in many forms, and it is wonderful to die away from things or situations that are no longer needed. We have refused to see that death can be positive and that what dies can make room for something better to live. Women have the greatest understanding of the connection to life and death through the blood of their bodies. Therefore, I believe one of women's key roles is to teach the importance of cycles and thereby steer us away from uniformity and consistency. We live in a political climate that spews dogma about respecting diversity, yet the diversity women bring from a biological level, the diversity that lives in every female, remains completely disregarded. We must allow and support the cycles that promote positive change in our lives. We must allow death to come to the emotions, beliefs, and situations that are no longer appropriate in our lives in order to create more harmonious and cooperative lives. If we can understand and respect how endemic cycles are to all of life, perhaps we can interact more as participants rather than controllers, allowing healing to occur from the inner wisdom directed through cycles of change.

LISTENING SONG
—Rebecca Smith Orleane

Tumbling Waters
Winds that roll across the sky,
Soaring Eagle,
Come to teach me how to fly.

I am listening,
Listening, listening for your cry.
I am listening,
Eagle, teach me how to fly.

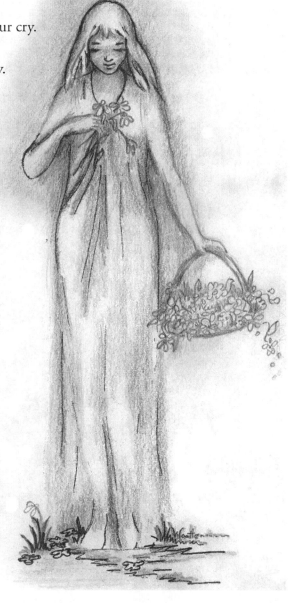

SEVEN:
DEEP LISTENING

On the Monday before Thanksgiving I awakened at dawn full of gratefulness for my heartmate, who was quietly sleeping beside me. I crept out of our bed and made my way to the kitchen table. As I grabbed my pen, all the many things he brings to our relationship were present in my heart and on my mind, and I just had to write them down. It's not that he had done anything unusual or out of character. I was just aware of who he is, and I was grateful.

I chose different colors of paper, representing all the ways he colors and brightens my life. Four days later, I was still thinking of more things about him for which I am thankful. On Thanksgiving dawn, I once again slid out of the covers and made my way to the kitchen to finish the love project I had begun. I cut out my list of "thank yous" and taped them to the walls all over our house: a "Thanksgiving" surprise for when he woke up.

After his delighted discovery, I went for a walk by myself in the snowy, quiet morning. I could feel the presence of my guardian angels, my guides, my spirit teachers, around me as I walked, something that I am frequently aware of when I stop to pay attention. This particular morning, they offered me their perfume, and I stood and marveled in the new morning snow at the gift of spiritual guidance exuding in an way that I could comprehend: the smell of flowers was all around me!

As I walked, my morning thoughts were a communication flowing back and forth between my guides and me. We had a conversation. Not the type of conversation between humans, nor the conversation of someone arguing with herself. No. I realized that they were placing understandings in my heart, and from these understandings, ideas rose into my head. I told them thank you for their presence and their help, and they gave me more perceptions. I was thinking from my heart, and I knew I was in the presence of divinity.

Each of us has our own belief about receiving spiritual help. Some of us believe in guardian angels or spirit teachers; some of us believe it comes from God; some of us believe it is the wisdom of our own intuition. I tend to interchange the terms guides and intuition, for I believe they are intimately connected. But whether we attribute the guidance we receive to our intuition, to guardian angels, to God, or to spirit teachers, we cannot hear it if we don't slow down and listen.

Listening, really listening, is a holy experience. It requires letting go of our preconceived notions about who and how we are. It requires willingness to be divine in order to connect with the divine. It requires getting out of our own way and accepting what comes to us as *real*, blessings that we deserve because we are spiritual beings, blessings that we can share with others through accepting our spiritual nature.

Understanding how spirituality is important within life's cycles involves knowing when to listen and when to speak. As dual biological beings, women *can* be wonderful examples of being good listeners and knowing when to speak. We know how to be good listeners. We listen to our children. We listen to our partners. We listen to our friends. Whether we are hearing a friend pour out of some deep secret, our lifemate share an important goal, or the small voice of a child's dreams, we know that listening can make a difference. We *have* to listen: it's in our blood. We also know that in order to *really* listen, we have to stop doing everything else and pay attention. It is only then that we get the depth of the sharing.

We have to stop doing and *listen* to hear the voice of our intuition or our guides as well. While we know that the best way to hear is to put aside the everyday chatter and clean out the personal emotional garbage that can confuse and interfere with our understanding, we are often "too busy" to simply stop and listen. Even when we understand that we *need* to slow down, we are pressured by the demands of our lives to such an extent that we often don't follow the soft voice of our inner wisdom telling us to slow down or stop.

Nature gives women a biological opportunity to slow down and listen so that we can hear what our guides, or our intuition, or our emotional wisdom, have to say. But culturally we have been programmed to put our own needs last in order to take care of others. Our culture resists our natural inclination to go inward, compelling us to busy ourselves taking care of others rather than valuing what we could receive from the deep listening that requires we put other duties aside.

The governing myths of our culture discount the necessity of retreating to honor our connection to unseen knowing and scorn women's "intuition" as superstition. Far too often we "have a feeling" about something or "just know" what needs to be done without being able to explain why. Without a rational explanation or scientific backing for our directions, our inner wisdom is discounted as unimportant or unreasonable. I am sure each of you can count times when you have "known" something and been lead to act (or not act) according to what you knew and have been talked out of it, or actually talked yourself out of it, only to look back and say "I knew better" or "I should have listened to my intuition."

The doctrine of feminism, which came about to help women be recognized as equals to men, has played a part in the suppression of our inner guidance, our own rhythms, and the suppression of menstruation itself. In the race to be seen and treated equally, a noble cause, we have laid aside the understanding that having a monthly cycle brings knowledge that men do not have, can never have. Radical feminists, seeking to compete with men, have insisted that women can do everything that men can do any time of the month. Of course we can. But *should* we???

Knowing when to speak and how to speak in a way that we can be heard has been more challenging for women in Western patriarchal cultures. Our voices have been silenced or ignored when we have been speaking our greatest truths. We have been dismissed far too often. Frequently the feminine need to be heard outweighs what a woman might have to say if she reached into her own heart and voiced her most important truths; what spills out is empty chatter and what needs to be voiced goes unsaid. Speaking too much about too little has caused an even greater dismissal by some of the very ones we long to have hear us the most. Because we have struggled so hard to be heard, many women have lost the balance of when to listen and when to speak. My heart aches when I see a woman who has found a doorway to being heard, and doesn't know when to close it. I silently watch many women engaging in empty chatter rather than speaking what lies dormant or unlistened to within their own hearts.

Every day I see hundreds of women on cell phones. They are talking while they drive, while they walk, while they shop.

I even saw one man kissing a woman while she was talking on her cell phone! Talk about a missed opportunity. I would certainly rather be totally present with the gift of a kiss than to absently receive it while I am reaching for connection through an impersonal cell phone.

Women are so hungry for connection and so desperate to be heard that some of us have forgotten that it is important to seek a balance in when to listen and when to speak. This imbalance cannot help but interfere with our spiritual listening as well. It is not enough to listen to our intuition when it is convenient, or listen for spiritual guidance only while we are in church, or to ask in prayer for the solutions to our problems without an equal amount of listening. Even in prayer, many of us have forgotten the balance between speaking (or asking) and listening (or receiving).

We have also forgotten the link between our deep listening and our sexuality. Deep listening within our sexuality is linked to our spirituality. Because sexuality has been demoted in our culture to a commodity and, like everything else in our linear society, is focused on progress and an end result (foreplay and an orgasm,) the deep listening (to our own bodies as well as to the hearts of our partners) required to make sexual exchange a spiritual experience is often lost, leaving many women asking why sex is worth it. Sex therapist Gina Ogden points to a "cultural taboo: the national terror of endowing our sensual, sexual pleasures with any measure of spiritual value" (13).

Emilie Conrad explains that in a phallic society a woman has tremendous power, so disempowering women is a way to retain male control.

If our sexual experiences are separated from our spiritual experiences in order to retain the current hierarchy of control, how can we achieve the full, wild abandon necessary for sex to be spiritual? If we are focused on "pleasing" or "being pleased", we are not listening to the call to surrender necessary for holy union. Christians refer to "the holy trinity" as "Father, Son, and Holy Ghost." I refer to the holy trinity, in sexual terms, as "Self, Loved-One, Divine." To join those three in the ecstasy of a spiritual-sexual union involves deep listening to Divinity and joining our own voices in the stream of bliss.

Politically, environmentally, and biologically it is easy to see how we may have become imbalanced in both our daily living and our spiritual lives, which by the way, are not separate and should not be treated separately. Too often what we speak is only what we know and feel from our own little worlds. If we don't detach from our own way of being, in order to listen and to change, we cannot offer anything of substance to our families or our world.

Even if we do not use our sacred cleanse to prepare for new life, retiring to listen to spiritual guidance brings greater harmony as a result of ideas, solutions, brainstorms, and inspiration that arrive through dreams. The portal to the spiritual realm is not as open at any other time as when we are in the flow of cleansing and preparation. At that time we need to be in our own space, free of distracting influences. If we are sleeping with someone else, (a non-menstruating woman or, particularly, with a man, whose energy is a polar opposite to the energy of Nature's gift,) this pure divine guidance can be confused with the presence of the person's energy or dreams; hence, we cannot be sure that what we receive is truly ours.

Finding a time to detach in retreat is important for all of us, and more important for women, who are biologically engineered to have a natural urge to slow down and listen. There is a right order in the timing of every day and what each day needs from us. Yet our calendar conscious culture dictates a meager space for rest ("week-ends" that are usually full of other responsibilities) that does not match our inner biological urgings to slow down at the right time. This artificial designated "rest period" is another indication of the many ways that we have divided ourselves from our spiritual nature every day.

With the introduction of electric lights, schedules, and more choices about whether or not to have children, women's bodies have sped up to keep pace with the complexities of modern life. At the same time, women have become more fragile, and are often more easily upset because we are so affected by the imbalances we face every day. There are many imbalances impinging on us: hormones in food, toxins in our air and water, too fast a pace, and the many demands from our outer environment that we choose to honor at the expense of our inner environmental needs.

Men are affected too. We humans are more sensitive emotionally and physically than we accept. Often we feel so trapped by the demands on us, or so inadequate to make appropriate changes that we simply look for ways to numb the pain...a glass of wine to soothe us or an escape through our favorite TV show: anything outside ourselves that can serve to distract us from what we feel and what we need to examine to make positive changes in our lives. Rarely do we stop to listen to see what our spiritual guidance or our intuition is asking. We just keep pushing forwards until we collapse into an exhausted sleep.

Lack of spiritual listening can contribute to misplaced anger, as well. Because we don't slow down to listen to what is wrong, we are not always appropriately angry at the right thing or the right person. More and more often we engage in the darker sides of human behavior, expressing inappropriate anger verbally, or even violently, out of frustration from not having our needs met or not taking steps to meet our own needs. I am horrified daily that violence has been accepted as a normal part of life.

Yet as imbalanced as modern life has become, there are avenues open for change, if we only allow time to listen to our spiritual guidance. As life has become more complicated, Nature has compensated, giving women more cycles of bleeding than our ancestors had, more chances to bring our lives into balance and to lead our families towards balance. But when we don't honor this natural time for slowing down to listen, we miss the guidance cues we have been given.

In this modern age of extreme imbalances, it is even more important for women to use their monthly cycles as opportunities for rebalancing. We need to rest, to listen to our inner guidance, and to act on the wisdom we receive in our hearts from listening. The faster the world moves, the more we have become out of sync with Nature. It is our sacred responsibility to live in harmony with Nature and to teach by example how to do that. If we don't, our loved ones, our children, and we ourselves are doomed.

There is a connection to spirituality and the sacred ability to bring life into the world. Women possess this most sacred of gifts; we are life givers. When we are biologically preparing for the possibility of performing this awesome task, we have the greatest opportunity for deep listening. It is during our bleeding cycles that we have the chance and the duty to move into a sacred realm for deeper connection to Source: to *listen*. It is only when we listen that we can know what to do and how to do it.

If we insist on moving through our days as if they are all the same, continually "doing", we forfeit the gifts of simply "being". We don't dwell in the space of sacred listening. If we don't slow down to listen during the biological time we have been given for rebalancing, we imbalance ourselves by being too active, too full, to outspoken without the benefit of inner wisdom from listening to inner guidance.

To stay immersed in the mundane rather than to use our monthly cycles as an opportunity for greater connection with Source is profane. We simply *must* honor this powerful time of purification and preparation. Even if we do not create a life, deep listening during our bleeding allows God, Spirit, or our intuition to guide us in ways to create greater harmony, bringing us ideas, solutions, brainstorms, and inspiration though dreams and quiet listening. The portal to guidance is not as open at any other time as when we are in the flow of our bleeding cycles.

Jack Kornfield has eloquently expressed the appropriateness of personal retreats for spiritual insight:

"Just as there is beauty to be found in the changing of the earth's seasons and an inner grace in honoring the cycles of life, our spiritual practice will be in balance when we can sense the time that is appropriate for retreats" (14).

This idea pertains directly to the connection between deep listening and retreat at the right time; taking this further, retreat during Nature's gift is implicated as being significantly beneficial for women's spiritual experiences.

If women give themselves the experience of sleeping in their own space during menstruation (the time of cleansing, listening, and preparation) rather than sleeping with a man (who has polar opposite energy) or with a non-menstruating woman, they can be very clear about claiming the guidance they receive as theirs. If women combine their energy with others during this special time, pure divine guidance can become mixed and confused with the presence of other's dreams, leading them to question what is truly theirs.

Historically, indigenous women understood the connection between spirituality and the power available during the bleeding time of their cycles. Although women could not avoid physical and spiritual dangers brought on by menstruation and childbirth, they knew they could gain spiritual understanding and spiritual power at these times. In Cherokee culture, menstruation and childbirth were associated with spiritual power. Menstruating women in particular were considered to have great power, and men regarded them as dangerous; they were sacred *because* they were dangerous and dangerous *because* they were sacred.

Yurok grandmothers taught young women that the potential for spiritual accomplishment was brought by the power of menstrual blood. They believed that this special time should not be wasted in mundane tasks and social distractions. Instead, all a woman's energy should be invested in listening in order to accumulate spiritual energy and to understand what was required for their lives.

The Kolish Indians of Alaska confined pubescent girls in

a tiny hut, completely blocked except for one small air hole, for one year, during which time they were allowed no fire, no exercise, and no company. The Kolish believed that this type seclusion forced the young girl to go into a meditative state, since she could do nothing else. She learned how to listen to spiritual guidance and carried that wisdom with her for life.

The connection between spirituality and menstruation is missing in modern culture. Listening for intuitive or spiritual guidance during Nature's gift can bring information for a woman herself or information for a larger community. Some things that come during menstrual listening are *only* for the woman experiencing Nature's gift. She may act on her wisdom, but she would not share what she learned. Other things that may be heard are appropriate for bringing creative solutions back to the family or the community. Yet even if a woman is receiving private advice only for her own life, if she listens to and acts upon what her intuition or spiritual guidance offers, she can learn creative ways to re-balance her family and her community.

Harmony is contagious. When a woman has cleared herself from old blood, stale emotions, and negative energy, and she has listened well, she radiates a kind of peace and harmony that goes outward towards those around her. She comes out of the menstrual questing place, and as the moon moves from darker to light, she also begins to become full of light and energy to be used creatively for life.

As already discussed, the wisdom of biology supports ritual separation for women during Nature's gift. It is well recognized that women's hormones (FSH, LH, estrogen, and progesterone) all fluctuate monthly and are all low during menses. The relationship between biochemical lows and interpersonal non-attachment during a menstrual retreat may affect spiritual experiences. Also it is possible that the psychological break of time apart during menses may offer the opportunity to see things with a fresh perspective.

I am not suggesting that extreme seclusion is appropriate today, yet I want to again state that designated retreat time, whether sleeping alone or simply slowing down one's daily pace, have proven to be beneficial to women worldwide. I also want to reiterate that ritual seclusion practiced by women in indigenous cultures was consistently something chosen by women for women. It was not a cruel discipline forced on women by men, but rather an opportunity women *chose*, even as young girls, to deepen their understanding of the mystery of life.

The connection between spirituality and menstruation is missing in modern culture. In fact, the spiritual component has gone missing from most modern rituals, leaving a secular and insipid shell of what once were deeply meaningful rituals. We have retained graduation ceremonies and Church weddings, but even these are sometimes more a matter of form, lasting a very short time, rather than a designated lengthy time of real inward listening.

High school graduation exercises are all that remain of coming of age rituals for either gender. The idea of a coming of age ritual surrounding menstruation is foreign to our youth. Most American boys giggle at the idea of menstruation, and phrases such as "on the rag," "the curse," or "fell off the roof" have the effect of teaching girls that menstruation is negative and must be hidden. There is no modern day ritual to link a young menstruant with the honor of becoming a woman who can bring forth life.

Western culture has suppressed or denied women (and men) the understanding and the *honor* of most of our natural biological cycles, as the separation from Nature has occurred. We have not learned the value and benefit of using natural rhythms to clean out what isn't working, to listen for guidance, or to incubate new creative ideas. We have not been taught to honor menses as a time of the month when we are extremely receptive (to dreams, creative ideas, to processing what is not working). Slowing down to *receive* guidance is not considered as important as being productive in our culture. Listening has less value than speaking.

Spirituality and intuition are sisters. In fact, in many instances they are the same. Our intuition can arise from our body awareness, from patterns that our brains recognize, or from whispers and nudges from our guides, or guardian angels. Women have historically been recognized as intuitive creatures. Our "sixth sense" has been noted as a strange anonomoly, a scary phenomenon, or a gift from the gods. I believe intuition is a product of recognizing patterns held by the body or in our learned mental experience. I also believe that intuition is often a pure and simple result of our deep listening to the guides that are trying to help us. We absolutely must return to the matriarchal understanding of balance, and honoring menstruation as a ceremony and a necessary retreat is one way that we can reclaim and direct the use of the sacred power we carry in our blood. If we do this for ourselves, we do it for all humanity.

It is time women wake up and face the shadow of who we have become. We need to reach deeply inside to find our connection with guidance. We need to put aside our fear, face our shadows, and move towards our monthly opportunity to connect with natural wisdom. We carry the possibility of always hearing needed answers for our world by virtue of our innate biological connection to Nature. We are lightbeings; we are healers; we are spiritual guides for our world. It is time that we honor the timing of our own bodies and move into being who we really are.

While I have been insisting that special retreat during menstruation is appropriate and necessary for the opportunities it offers to listen to spiritual guidance, I do not believe that any one period of time is the *only* time we can connect to our guidance. In fact, I believe that the more we honor special times, the more spiritual guidance and intuition come to us on a daily basis.

I have long held the opinion that we should celebrate the sacredness of life every day, not just on calendar marked "special times." It is appropriate to set aside special times to share with loved ones, to decorate our homes, to prepare special food, and to honor the natural ceremony of menstruation.

The Western holiday of Thanksgiving is a good reminder to us to be thankful for all the goodness we have in our lives. Yet how many of us tell people thank you for who they are and what they do on a daily basis? A one-day holiday offering spiritual thanks is a good way to remind us to be spiritually thankful every day. In the same way, a monthly retreat of deep listening for guidance can remind us to listen as we move through our daily routines the rest of the time.

The man with whom I share my life practices expressing gratefulness on a daily basis. I have had the pleasure of hearing him thank me, thank checkout clerks, thank people on the phone, for every small kindness he receives. He also sets aside time on a regular basis to listen for guidance. He is a wonderful example of practicing gratefulness on an everyday basis, and I understand from living with him that being in a state of thankfulness and wonder keeps the flow of harmony going. It just doesn't stop. We also share the understanding of the importance of slowing down to listen at regular intervals.

The importance of bleeding cycles for clearing, then creating life can be extended to the understanding of human breath cycles. Regardless of our spiritual beliefs, we cannot breathe without accepting the gift of life. We can breathe in life and divinity, and we breathe out our own energy to others as either unconditional acceptance and love or negative judgments. We have the same opportunity to honor our cycles and be careful of what we release through our breathing as we do when we are releasing our blood. We are all part of the cycle of life. We give back to life by breathing out what we have breathed in. Giving and receiving. Receiving and giving. Let us honor the connections between breath cycles, blood cycles, and life, and let us be careful in how we engage with them. As women, it is our sacred duty to teach the importance of honoring cycles through the example of how we live our lives.

THE HEART OF RELATIONSHIP
—Rebecca Smith Orleane

It is in the heart

That all differences

Can move into Unity.

Begin a loving relationship with yourself,

And you will find loving relationships with others.

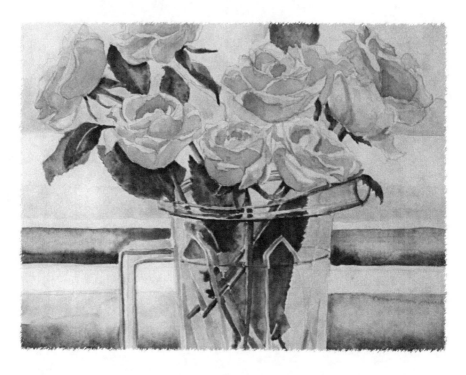

EIGHT:

RELATIONSHIPS OF THE HEART

After I freed myself from the prison of my second marriage, it was several years before I met my heartmate. I knew instinctively that I must create a better relationship with myself before I was going to manifest a kind and loving relationship with anyone else, and so I spent those years in a committed relationship with *myself*. I learned to ask the right questions and to listen to the answers my heart whispered (or sometimes shouted) to me. Who was I? What were my gifts? What did I need? What fears did I need to work through and release? What dreams guided me on my path? And so I journeyed through the heart, asking for guidance and listening to what it had to say.

I had fired my second husband for an inability to see who I was and for failure to meet me on any level. When I left him standing in shocked disbelief, he did his utmost to color me through outright lies. Even thinking about another relationship made me realize that I was frightened of having another person try to steal my spirit, disempower me, override my needs with his own agenda, or disrespect me. I had good reason to be shell-shocked about relationships; I had been badly bruised by disrespect, and I was determined to respect myself enough to never allow that to happen again. I will share with you what I discovered as I journeyed away from fear towards love.

To start the discovery of relationship awareness, I must begin at the core. To see to the heart of relationships, we must begin with the relationship we have with ourselves. A man in couples therapy in my office once asked his wife, "Do you love me better than anybody else?" From the content of their discussion, I knew he was not referring to other men, or even family and friends. He was asking for her to love him best because he did not love himself. I knew she had done her own work when she responded, "Of course not. I have to love myself before I can love anyone else." That kind of spontaneous answer comes from the high self-esteem required for love to blossom.

My entire philosophy about love is based on my understanding that if a woman does not love herself, does not see the wonder of who she is, she will forever be doomed to searching for that special look in the eyes of another. (The same applies to men.) On the other hand, if a woman loves herself and accepts her imperfections as part of who she is, there is room for her to invite another in to share love in relationship.

I believe women's failure to love themselves, reflected as low self-esteem, is one large part of so many failed relationships. (This is true for men, too.) How can anyone *else* supply a person with self-esteem? Self-esteem must come from inside. It must come from accepting who we are and loving ourselves totally, blemishes and beauty alike. For women in a patriarchal society, it is even more imperative to love ourselves first. We simply must stop looking to men (or anyone else) to fill that place of knowing that we are glorious beings. Relying on someone else to value you is a recipe for disaster in relationship.

While it is narcissistic to love *only* yourself, it is not narcissistic to love yourself *first*. In fact it is absolutely *necessary* to love and truly value yourself before you can truly love and value another. Airline attendants always instruct passengers to put the oxygen on oneself before helping small children. That's because if you don't take care to get the oxygen you need, you will pass out and be *unable* to help a child. The same logic applies to loving yourself. If you don't give yourself the love and acceptance you need, valuing both your talents and your wounded places, you will not be able to truly value and love another. You will, instead, do the equivalent of passing out from lack of oxygen. Passing out from lack of self-love and self-regard causes one to shrink away from wholeness, to become dependent on external forces to supply what is needed.

That's right. You start believing that the beloved is responsible for your self-esteem and for providing the experience of being loved. That's all wrong. The *feeling* of being loved is an *internal* state, and it is our responsibility to foster that within ourselves by loving ourselves.

The ability to love another is born out of an internal state of loving, having so much love present, it naturally wants to be shared with another. If there is a dearth of self-love and warm self-regard, we quite naturally as humans, seek to fill the need. Movies, advertising, and cultural myths have incorrectly instructed us that we can get that need filled from the love of another. Our culture supports the illusion of romantic longing for the one who can fill the emptiness, that special someone who can become our "other half." I recommend that if you want a healthy relationship, you look for someone who can be your "other *whole*" and who supports your being whole yourself.

Relationship is one of women's sacred interests. Yet cultural assumptions and false advertising have tarnished our view of relationship. Marketing and cheap movies have lead women (and many men) on a wild goose chase of romantic notions that have little to do with deep relationship or real love. Many women believe that they must cast their nets to capture the essence of love. That perspective only leads to getting tangled in the line. Sexy clothes and sweet smelling perfumes will not draw a man of honor to our sides. While most men appreciate beauty and sweetness, a man of deep character will not be won through artificial tricks, at least not for long.

Sexuality has been deeply tarnished in our culture. Media throws sex into our face to sell cars or vegetables, while religion takes the stance that sex is appropriate only under the guidelines of the Church. Women today are often confused, feeling they are lacking if they don't have active sex lives and are condemned if they do. It is not the focus of this book to address that issue, yet it is so deeply important to what is out of balance, that I must say something, if only peripherally.

There is a joke that says "men talk to women in order to have sex, and women have sex in order to talk to men." Sadly, there is some truth in that. Many women today engage in sex in an effort to find intimacy and connection. But that is painfully backwards! In the most common misunderstanding, modern men and women link sex to intimacy and actually believe that if they are having sex, they are being intimate. That, of course, is ideal, but sadly, it is far from true. Intimacy and sex are not the same thing. Sex *can* come from intimacy, but is not necessarily intimate. Intimacy is being completely comfortable with being who you are in the presence of the other person. Why would you share your body with someone whom you do not feel like you can completely be yourself? We need to address our assumptions about intimacy and sexuality to understand the importance of exploring true intimacy before we explore sexuality, for sex without intimacy is shallow and sad and often focuses only on performance, not connection. Sex therapist Gina Ogden points out that performance sex tends to bypass our feelings and the meanings attached to sexual sharing. She says, "it bypasses our deep connections with the rhythms of the planet"(15). Need I say more?

We need more *connection*, not more sex. I believe the reason so many women love to dance and bemoan the fact that they can't get their partners to dance with them is because they are seeking connection. Shuttle and Redgrove point out that the accented rhythms of dance play an important part in "activating the feminine style of conscious, as it puts women in touch with their own body rhythms"(16). Dancing is a way of reaching out to another person and sharing each other's rhythms. Women inviting their partners to dance are offering to share their life rhythms with them. I believe men are who are afraid to dance are often afraid they will perform poorly. What they fail to realize is that the best performance they could achieve has very little to do with proper dance steps. It has to do with the act of sharing your partner's rhythm and your rhythm with her, and by sharing rhythms, achieving true connection.

The current "romantic" model for relationships actually contributes to co-dependent thinking in relationships and may, quite possibly, foster increased divorce rates. It is impossible for an external source (the beloved partner) to continuously provide the necessary stream of love endorphins we need for our own self-regard, and it is exhausting for them to try. Think of how tiring it is to continually try to make someone else happy who is unable to access his own inner happiness. It is an unfair request to anyone we truly value and love, for the other person cannot attend to his own internal needs and rewards if he constantly has to monitor ours. How can that be a balanced relationship of any duration? Of course the divorce rate goes up. Emotional exhaustion and lack of self growth lead both partners to either resign themselves to less than they deserve, or to look for another source to supply the "high" of being in love.

In a healthy relationship, each person attends to her own internal states, refilling the well of love so that there is more to drink from and to offer. Many women fall into the trap of looking for romantic love and the idealization of themselves through their lover's vision. Cultural messages encourage this misshapen thinking. Movies, television, magazine ads project skinny models who parrot the cultural imperative that women must be perfect and constant to be loved. It is no small wonder that having a monthly cycle, with its accompanying look at what is wrong in a woman's life has become so unaccepted. In our culture, there is no room to examine places that reflect our shadow, places where we long for change and improvement. Simple acceptance of this aspect of our femininity would increase our self-esteem and enhance our influence enormously. If women valued their insights that arise during this powerful time, and were applauded for the creative solutions that arise from dark internal places, perhaps we could break the vicious pattern of needing to be continually perfect, or perfect at all.

The myth of perfection extends from our own inadequacies outward to damage our relationships as well. We have been led to believe that if we are perfect, we are capable of finding "Mr. Right" and making a perfect relationship. What flawed thinking! Our views of perfection have become rigidly determined by an artificial value system, with no sense of flow or opportunity for change. Mistakes are not often seen in our culture as something to be accepted as an avenue for growth. We make a mistake, and we *learn* from it. Our partner makes a mistake, and he *learns* from it. Together we grow.

Our society has romanticized the notion of partnership and marriage to such an extent that once we are in the glow of new love, women (and men) often make an unhealthy leap in assumption that it will always be that way, if they have found the right person. (I rarely hear people in my therapy practice asking if they *are* the right person.) The fairy tale mentality that says, "and they lived happily ever after" keeps both genders looking for "Mr. or Ms. Right".

Because of our societal emphasis on constancy, couples find themselves baffled at the natural cycles present in relationship. Like everything in life, there are times of sharing and times to do things on our own. There are times that we are clicking on all cylinders and can share what we are thinking with just a glance, and times when every word we utter seems to be misconstrued. Suddenly discovering that relationships, like everything else, have cycles, leads many couples to question if they have the right partner. This is probably the most important place that women could share an understanding of how everything cycles from their own biological wisdom, if only they would heed that voice. In a society that seeks and promotes constancy and fairy tales that end with "and they lived happily ever after," we have all been lead down a fantasy trail that not only does not exist, but would be boring if it did! I would love to hear the fairy tale that ended with "And they continued to grow and change for the rest of their days!"

Unfortunately, too many of us in the bliss of new love, fall into believing that our loved one is perfect, only to be sorely disappointed when he makes a little mistake. It follows also, that if we expect our mate to be perfect, we want to be seen as perfect ourselves (like the Hollywood models we imitate.) So when *we* make a mistake (or move into the dark phase of our cycle to wrestle with our own psyche), our self-esteem drops and we struggle to accept love being offered, for we do not, at that moment, love ourselves.

It is dangerous to desire perfection within ourselves or to project that the person with whom we are mated is perfect, although they may indeed be the perfect partner *for us*. Trying to be perfect does not allow room for the mistakes from which we grow. Telling someone else that they are perfect assigns them the task of having to live up to *being* perfect. How tiring. And what a time bomb for conflict. Perfection for one person is flawed for another. The tension of demanding perfection in ourselves or in our mates leads to huge disappointments and potential conflict, internally and externally.

Good relationships are born out of understanding that we are connected even when we disagree; we must respect our differences as well as our likenesses. No one way of being human is perfect, and the beauty of our differences is what causes attraction to begin with. We are all parts of one human family, one body, like drops of water in the same ocean. Approaching relationship from this angle allows each of us to be imperfect beings moving towards our higher selves. With the one special person we choose, the one who is *not perfect,* but perfect *for us,* we can work from a mutually shared worldview to help each other grow.

One of the most important ingredients for success in any relationship is being able to disagree, or if necessary, fight fairly. The conflicts in which we engage from our differing points of view become the fodder for our growth. If fighting is necessary (and sometimes it is), it is imperative to be an honorable warrior, lest you injure the person and relationship you hold most dear. It is important to know how to be fight with integrity. I have a formula for fighting with honor and integrity.

First, we must *recognize the enemy*. That seems obvious, but it isn't always so apparent when we are in the middle of confusing emotions. While sometimes the enemy actually *is* the person standing in front of us (as in abusive or narcissistic relationships), more often the enemy is the misunderstanding between us. In healthy relationships, the enemy is the discord, not the person. To restore harmony, the place of discord must be determined, and each person must be allowed to fully express his or her viewpoint without judgment or blame.

The second ingredient for fighting with integrity is *compassion*. It is *absolutely* necessary to be compassionate in the middle of battle in order to respect each person's integrity and to preserve the relationship. We must have compassion for ourselves and what we are feeling, *and* have compassion for the other's feelings. Compassion does not mean that you give in to the other side. It is a simple acknowledgment that the other person must be feeling some discomfort, distress, or emotional pain, or they would not be doing what they are doing or saying what they are saying. Compassion requires listening with an open heart, sharing with an open heart, and not reacting to what is heard or shared. In the midst of disagreement, it helps to not only listen to the other point of view, but to also sense the other person's pain. Acting and reacting with compassion allows your heart to release its grip of anger and soften towards resolution.

The third ingredient is *strength*. Being strong is not the same as being obstinate. There is gentleness in real strength, as any "gentle-man" will show you. Being strong is recognizing when to insist on being heard, and when to yield to listening. In the cycle of an argument, there is a space for both. If you find it is not possible to do both, it is not a fair fight. Fighting with integrity requires combining gentleness with strength and refusing to forfeit one for the other.

A fourth ingredient I encourage is *paying attention to your mantra*. (A mantra is an idea that is repeated, often without thinking about it). What are we saying about ourselves or about the other person when we are in the heat of battle? Continually repeating to yourself "He is such a jerk!" is not a helpful mantra. It is merely an expression of your frustration, and continually repeating it only further assigns your partner the role you expect him to play. I find it helpful to have a positive mantra in my head, something like "I know I can say what I need to with kindness," or "I know he wants to understand me," or "I know my heartmate loves and respects me even if we disagree." An effective mantra removes you from the carnage of battle and keeps you steady on your path as an honorable warrior.

I have suggested mantras to clients when they have been going through difficult situations. For someone who continually feels accountable for other people's behavior, the mantra, *"I am not responsible for his bad choices"* works really well. When a client is overly concerned about what others say about them, I suggest trying, *"what he thinks (or says) about me is none of my business!"* I have offered this mantra to clients undergoing difficult relationship splits; it helps to defuse hurtful rumors and outright lies.

A fourth important ingredient for healthy disagreements is to the value of *timing*. Military leaders use timing to look for advantage, a chance to take the enemy off guard. This type of timing does not work for relationship issues. (Remember, the enemy is the misunderstanding, not the person). A person fighting with honor and integrity *looks for an opportunity to bring resolution.* Fighting with honor is not about proving your point or making the other person wrong. Fighting with honor disallows name-calling or belittling remarks. Fighting with honor requires that you preserve the integrity of the other's self-esteem during the battle, not destroy it with your "justified" emotional outbursts. Timing in battle is important. It is not the time to engage in battle when one partner is feeling down or discouraged. Nor is it good timing to blast our mate with our viewpoint when we are overwrought with emotion. It is kinder in both situations to say, *"let's discuss this later,"* or *"I am too angry (or hurt) to talk about this right now. Can we discuss it in a few hours (or tomorrow)?"* Honoring the right timing to resolve a disagreement is one of the ways we can respect cycles in relationship. There is a time for everything, and being flexible to allow the right timing to unfold creates greater opportunities for harmony.

These four ingredients for honorable arguments within personal relationships can be applied to all relationships; the key for making the formula work is that *both* partners must play by the rules of fair fighting, and *both* must act with inscrutable integrity. If both partners don't play by the rules, there will be wounds that may be difficult to heal or relationship carnage. Asking for forgiveness later may be too late.

Integrity in relationship requires being who you are in the face of adversity. That means not caving in out of guilt at your own imperfections, nor being angry at another for what you perceive as their imperfections. Proper timing in addressing conflict is enhanced by the idea of withdrawing during emotional flags that may arise during your cycle in order to assess what needs to occur. This type of emotional assessment keeps irritating issues from building to a point of insurmountable conflict. The indigenous idea of separation during menses creates a natural rhythm of withdrawing and coming together within our relationships. We not only protect the relationship from harmful emotions that need to be processed first within ourselves, we also gain the opportunity of deeper insight and creative ideas of how to do things differently. Withdrawing on a regular basis gives us a chance to face our difficulties authentically, calmly, and with compassion at the right time. When we do this, we love with all our heart, in a genuine manner. I believe the relationships of women who are still experiencing menstrual cycles benefit greatly from women employing a ritual that allows time and space for examination of one's own feelings first, and then the relationship.

Being in relationship gives us the chance to test what we have learned when we are by ourselves. It gives us opportunity after opportunity to live in challenging circumstances and move past our own fears and our own shadows. For really, whenever we are unhappy emotionally, a very big part of that emotion is a reflection of how we see ourselves, and what we carry from how others have reflected what they see of us.

Sometimes the choice of being true to ourselves overrides the choice of being in a particular relationship. When one is wounded from a relationship breakup, it is the perfect time to withdraw and examine what you want and to make some conscious choices about your life. Most people focus on what they *don't* want when they are recovering from a breakup, and that is part of the process. But only *part* of the process. The larger, often overlooked part is to determine what one *does* want.

Out of curiosity, I took a poll from my women friends, asking, "What is the number one most important thing in relationship to you?" Below are the reported requirements, in order of popularity of response:

- Trust
- Compatibility
- Honesty
- Respect
- Acceptance
- Having his own identity
- Being an Adult

It is interesting to me that none of them named Love. It seems to me that many women have given up on love as the basis of relationship, perhaps because of cultural definitions of romantic love or misunderstanding of what love is. Of course love can grow from trust and respect, as in arranged matches, or from friendships that develop into personal relationships, but certainly I believe love must be present for a successful relationship. For without love, the very heart of the relationship is missing. Without love, the heart is not open to sharing. Without love, all the other shining attributes pale.

Another important thing is missing from the above list, too. Passion. What's wrong with passion in your ideal relationship? Why is it that women have settled for passionless relationships in order to get other needs met? Personally, I want it all! And luckily, after two mistaken choices, I have a relationship that grants me that wish.

So often women (and men) hurry from one relationship to the next, in a desperate search for love or companionship. People leave out the necessary part of the cycle that allows for introspection and examination of what we have to offer and what we require. Just as modern day women ignore the introspective, quiet time of their bleeding cycles, they also ignore the dark times of aloneness. How can we know who we are or what we need, if we don't take the time to listen to what we have learned from one relationship before running headlong into the next?

I am a strong proponent of taking that time to build an even stronger relationship with yourself before you seek a relationship with another. It is important to explore your dreams, your desires, and your absolutely necessary requirements before you enter your next relationship. Often, out of hurt and loneliness, women (and men) skip this important step of investigation and move directly into the next relationship, building on the sand of "hope" that it will be better, rather than building on a firmer foundation.

I believe it is important for each of us to take time to really look at what we have learned from interactions in previous relationships. Very likely a woman is not the same person at the end of the relationship as she was at the beginning, and often she must heal a few wounds as well as to assess her strengths. Once she has done a thorough inventory of her own internal states, attributes, and desires, she can then spend some time listing what she wants in her next relationship. What is essential to her happiness and for her to thrive? What makes her laugh? What makes her feel safe? How does she recognize that she is being respected? What makes her feel both accepted and special? Once she has the answers to these questions, she can look for these traits in the people she considers, rather than trying to romanticize them into place in the throes of passion.

An important step in choosing the right partner for you is to examine that person's worldview. The predictive value of success in a relationship requires that both partners hold a similar worldview. That means that you share the same values, same priorities, same expectations and assumptions about life. Within that worldview there is lots of room for *individual* differences, goals, and opinions. That's what makes the relationship interesting! Carbon copy opinions are not what we are going after here. What we are going after is the ability to *respect* differences within the relationship while sharing the same global view on important issues (including spiritual beliefs, money and time management, views about children, etc.)

My own personal list of absolute essentials for relationship was devised during lengthy times of retreat for self-exploration and examination. These are the things that are necessary for *me* in relationship. Each woman should have her own list of requisites, but in my opinion, if the list doesn't start with *respect* as number one, you had better re-examine your list. Lack of respect for women is so endemic in our culture, women often fail to see that it is missing in the ardor of being pursued. When the roses arrive and the words are smooth and silky, desire for connection often overrules the warnings we might otherwise notice. Two more values that should head any list are *honesty* and *communication*. A relationship won't go far without these three. If you are evaluating a potential partner, notice how he treats others (check out clerks, friends, other women, siblings, business partners; Does he show road rage? Is he kind to animals?) How he treats others may be an important clue to how he will treat *you*. When you are listening to sweet whisperings in your ear, you had better open your eyes to see if his values are "lived" and real or "imagined" in his own head (or yours).

I consciously retreated to examine who I was, what I had learned, and what I had to offer, as well as what I wanted in relationship. I took my time, and thoughtfully, soulfully created my list. A year after my list was made, my ideal partner appeared, and we now joyfully share the loving relationship I searched for all my life! I met him at an art gallery. It was so obvious to me that he was special and different that I invited him to go on a walk. When he immediately said yes, I was surprised. We sat under a new moon and talked, and, while I was scared to acknowledge what my heart was telling me, inside *I knew* there was something extraordinary between us. My dreams had told me he was there, and I had hidden my head in the sand, refusing to look up. While I dragged my feet (failing to give him my phone number through months of letter writing), slowly my heart let go its fear and moved towards accepting love. Eventually I was ready to accept the gift I was being given. We moved quickly and flawlessly into relationship with each other, with a shared commitment to our divine growth and evolution.

I can honestly say, our relationship is deeply spiritual, deeply connective, passionate and fun, and it is obvious that we were meant to be together. If I had to go through all the lessons I endured (and apparently I did), life with my heartmate makes it worth it. So with this story as inspiration, I share below the list I came up with years ago. Bear in mind, please, that **Love** is the penultimate quality required for all relationships, in my opinion. But before love blooms, while it is blossoming, look for these:

- **Respect**
- **Honesty**
- **Communication** (two way- listening and speaking; being direct with kindness; clarity);
- **Trust** (if you can't trust him, how can you ever believe him? How can you share yourself with him?)
- **Kindness** (not just to you, to all of life)
- **Compassion**
- **Integrity**
- **Strength of character**
- **Generosity of spirit, time, and possessions**

- Loyalty and Devotion
- Confidence in himself
- Confidence in me
- Willingness to learn from me
- Willingness to teach me
- Understanding
- Acceptance (even when he doesn't understand)
- Good Boundaries balanced with appropriate sharing
- Concern for the Environment
- Desire to make a difference, service to others
- Desire to explore sexuality as a deeper form of connection and communication
- Ability to know himself
- Desire to grow and change
- Courage to grow and change
- Ability and desire to support *my* growth and change
- Love of Nature
- Love of music and beauty
- Love of silence
- Sense of Humor
- Ability to follow his own interests
- Willingness to explore activities with me
- Wise balance about when to put himself first and when to put me first

- **Independence balanced with desire to share**
- **Willingness to compromise**
- **Ability to discuss problems respectfully**
- **Health Consciousness**
- **Sensitivity to Timing**
- **Shared World View (including spiritual beliefs, assumptions, expectations, basic politics, and how to handle problems.)**

The last things on my original list were that I wanted my man to have the **ability to laugh at himself, at circumstances, and at life.** I wanted him to have **the soul of an Artist:** seeing the beauty of the world and loving it with passion. Obviously, if we could share all these things, we would enjoy each other's company. The last requirement that was essential for me was that my partner **cherish me and our relationship**. If these essentials were in place, and I matched them in giving, our love would be exquisite. I am happy to report, readers, that I did my work, and all my wishes came true.

Relationships are important to women (and to men.) Just take a look at any women's magazine today and you will see that relationship is still the number one area of women's interest. From deep within our bodies, women understand connection, and through that understanding, we often focus on relationships. With women's natural interest in relationships comes our sacred task to tend to relationships. Not that by any stretch we should *ever* take the sole responsibility for *any* relationship, but we must recognized with our natural feminine inclination to share our hearts comes the urge to guide the growth of our connections.

Relationships require effort. If someone in a relationship says, "My relationship is not working," unless the relationship is truly inappropriate, there is an implication that *someone* is not willing to do the required work of tending to the relationship. Relationships are like plants that need water, sunshine, and light. *And* as I have already said, they have cycles, just like plants and every other living thing.

Cycles in relationships dictate a time to come together and a time when he needs to go work on a project so you can breathe! I say this in humor because humor often holds the truth in a light way so we can look at it. The truth is that every partnership needs space- a time of separation and a time of union. Nature's gift is Nature's natural time for separation in relationships. It is a woman's own time, and the cold, moist, clearing energy during that time does not mix with hot, fiery, progress-oriented male energy. Sometimes it just these simple differences, without any external ruffle in the relationship, that cause men and women to psychically feel that they need to be apart.

Women and men are considered to have oppositional powers in many indigenous tribes, such as the Cherokee, the Yurok, the Dine, and the Apache. Oppositional powers are not considered positive versus negative, but simply different, like cold versus hot. The principle of opposite powers is obvious when one looks at Nature. Everything in Nature has an opposite: cold and hot, day and night, summer and winter. In many indigenous belief systems, women are considered cold and men hot. The extra cold (and wet) of a woman's menstrual cycle can put out the hot (and dry) fire of a man's energy. Indigenous women knew that they were so powerful they could potentially overwhelm male power; they chose to stay away from men during Nature's gift so as not to harm their men's opposite powers. St. Pierre and Long Soldier express the principle of opposites like this:

"A woman is the only one who can bring a child into this world. It is the most sacred and powerful of all mysteries. When a woman is having her time, her blood is flowing, and this blood is full of the mysterious powers that are related to childbearing. At this time she is particularly powerful. To bring a child into this world is the most powerful thing in creation. A man's power is nothing compared to this, and he can do nothing compared to it. We respect that power. You see, a woman's power and a man's are opposites-- not in a bad way, but in a good way. Because of the power a woman has during this time, it is best that, out of respect for her men, she stay away from them. In the past they would build a little lodge for her, and their other female relatives would serve on her needs.

She would get a rest from all her chores. It was not a negative thing like people think now. We did this out of respect for this great mystery, out of respect for the special powers of women" (17).

Encouraging time for a woman to listen to her body's wisdom keeps her from being locked into bad choices and allows her to move forward with positive change. It is incredibly important in relationships to honor the wisdom of the body's knowing, and setting aside Nature's gift as a time of deep listening encourages our inner wisdom to come forth. Nature's gift separation (and ritual separation for post-menopausal women) is a wonderful way to clean out incorrect assumptions, neediness, as well as hurts, anger, and depression. Withdrawing to do this while nurturing ourselves helps us to replenish the well so that we can come back to our respective relationships full again- full of love, positive self-regard, respect for others, creative ideas, and ability to offer ourselves for service to community. If we don't allow ourselves this opportunity, we can become trapped by choices we make without the value of deep listening.

The attempt to control when we bleed (or how much), the desire to follow cultural directions to treat every day the same (systemic homogenation) rather than honoring our dual natures, the total disregard and lack of understanding of the reasons for cycles, have caused women to devalue, ignore, hate, or dismiss one of Nature's most beautiful and valuable gifts. What should be a time of sensitivity and increased intuition for a woman in tune with the cycling of her own body, can become a well of sadness and misdirected anger within her relationships if she does not pay attention to what is not working and *listen* for guidance on how to change it. Yes, there are times when tears are appropriate. Tears are cleansing and can help to clear out problems and lubricate the way for solutions, but tears should be directly related to going inward and compassionately looking at our lives to see what is wrong, releasing the hurt and healing the situation. Tears should cleanse the way for intuitive spiritual guidance to bring us a creative solution. Out of the cleansing comes the direction we are to take. Tears are not supposed to be a source of guilt or shame because we are upset and frustrated. We are *not meant* to feel guilty because we are emotional or to be sad and not know why. Strong emotions are signposts to be used, not to be stuck away and hidden. Use emotions to recognize and be sensitive to what is out of balance. Grieve what is wrong, cleanse the way for change, and emerge from the experience clearer, better able to find another way.

The same goes for anger. There are times when it is appropriate to be angry. We should be angry about injustice, and we should take our anger to our sacred place where it can burn through the darkness of the injustice to reach the creative fire that brings change. Use your cycle, not to temper or control your anger, but to channel it to needed directions, to transform the raw emotion into strong, powerful action for change, for improving yourself, your relationships, your community. Use your anger to *make a difference.*

Once in a counseling session, a woman told me her story through tears of realization. She poured out words that had been stuffed inside of her for such a long time they could no longer be contained. She was trapped in an unhappy marriage she had chosen out of guilt. Angrily she told me,

> "For thirty-six years I have been married to the wrong man. I was 17 and I knew what was right and what was not. I started having asthma when he was around. My body told me to break up with him. When we were dating, I let my guard down, and he touched me when my body didn't want him to. I knew better. I had warning signs, but I didn't listen. I felt guilty because he touched me inappropriately, and I let him. I knew better, but I didn't stop him. I felt so guilty that I married him. Thirty-six years later, no matter how hard I try, I can't get him to listen to what is important to me. I should have listened to my own inner feelings."

She spilled her sorrow, like a swollen river, climbing out of its carefully held banks. This client is a tragic example of a woman who did not listen to the messages of her body, found herself locked into an unhappy relationship for her entire adult life, and did not know she had the power to change it.

Once again we are back to issue of valuing change, whether it is within our relationships as we pull apart and together again, or whether it is in our bodies to guide us through the different ways of being. Our indigenous elders knew that change, was the secret of life. Navajo women call the Creator of Life "Changing Woman" because she changes time and time again. Women elders taught that recognizing and honoring that changing nature inherent in women, the change that connected them to Nature through their cycles of bleeding, affected *all* relationships in a positive way. Therefore, they created the time of separation for women to honor the changes that come, the lifting of the veil between realities to allow better sight, the opportunity to grieve and get angry without having those emotions create toxicity in their relationships. The moon lodge, ritual separation, was a time to honor the emotions that rise to show us the way and tend to what needs fixing in our lives.

In my doctoral research, I interviewed men whose partners had agreed to separate sleeping during their cycles. I wanted to know what the men experienced from their mates' withdrawal once a month. Most shared with me that when their partners started using Nature's gift as a private time for introspection, they as a couple, learned how to fight in a healthier way. One man said to me, "Now I know why she has been mad at me for the last 17 years." Women often avoid conflict because of an intense desire for harmony; there is a fear that expressing dissatisfaction will cause such disequilibrium in the relationship that it will never recover, and may actually be lost. Sometimes this happens. But more often women's fear of conflict promotes suppression of (or mere whispering about) what is not working. When this happens a woman's dissatisfaction or her longing leak out in other ways that can poison the very relationship she holds dear. Having a ritual separation offers an opportunity for her to let the emotions of anger and sadness emerge in a safe way, a chance to really *sit* with her feelings until they are emptied. Once emptied of the negative emotions, something else can come in- something mystical and wonderful- guidance towards what she can do next and how to do it.

One thing we have not addressed is the aspect of forgiveness in relationships. It takes a loving heart to forgive, and it takes complete honesty and compassion with ourselves and with our mate to be able to forgive. We must accept that our little mistakes (and some of our big ones) are teaching tools to make us better human beings. We must be gentle with ourselves and equally gentle with our loved one when either of us makes a mistake. In a healthy, loving relationship, neither partner ever *intends* to hurt the other, yet we make mistakes just the same. Repeated mistakes often give us different vantage points of the challenge until we understand how to do it differently. It's how we grow.

Frequently we get our feelings hurt because we are fearful that our loved one does not love us enough or the right way, *"or else he wouldn't have done (or said) that."* We must move from fear of being hurt to trust that we are loved. Only the love is real. It is helpful to remember that our partner does not mean to hurt us when he says or does something that doesn't match our hopes or expectations. It is also helpful to be clear about our own actions so that we do the best we can in every moment. And we must always remember the rules of honorable fighting. If we live our lives like this, there is usually very little to forgive.

Before I close this chapter, I have few special things to say about relationship with children. Sometimes as parents women follow a path of trying to mold them- our girl children and our boy children- into "good human beings." It is almost as if each mother has taken a pledge by giving birth (or adopting) to invest herself in the outcome of her sacred trust. She comes to think that the special relationship she has with her child reflects her skills as a mother and her worth as a human being. I would like to encourage all mothers to understand that the sacred trust does not dictate that you mold your children. Rather, it is yours to shape the relationship by giving them a safe container in which to grown into Who They Are. If you guide them in the skills of being in relationship (with you, with friends, with the Earth, with all of life) and help them to understand that relationships have cycles as do all living things, you will have given them the greatest gift possible besides your love. Although most of this chapter has been aimed at intimate relationships, very likely you will find that *all* relationships flourish by following the same guidelines. Respect, honesty, communication, kindness, compassion, integrity, and a little laughter along the way. Are these not values that we want to use in relationship with our children, our friends, even in relationship with Mother Earth? The goal of this chapter has been to teach you a different way of being in relationship with every person, tree, or stone with which you come in contact, to become alive to being in relationship in every moment. We can facilitate healing our relationships and helping them grow through fully understanding that relationships are living things with cycles of their own.

A real honoring of the cyclic duality of life, for as long as we are experiencing dual nature, *may* automatically move into a cosmic spiral of greater unity, greater connection, and greater opportunities of creative life to blossom. Creativity in love is a wonderful gift. Spirals from cycles. Not polar opposites pushing against each other expressing the conflict of duality, but rather cycles spiraling closer and closer together to experience a wider array of possibilities. *This* is why women have cycles. To invite possibility. *This* is why women are so often peacemakers and caregivers, and why men who are also peacemakers and caregivers, carry so much feminine energy.

There is a knowing that movement (down and up, around and around) brings understanding, resolution, possibility: peace, peace, peace.

FIRST SNOW
—Rebecca Smith Orleane

Autumn whispers

   Hints of snow.

   Clouds descend on Mountain

  Pressing up to meet Source.

   I, too, prepare myself,

Moving quietly towards

    Depths of winter.

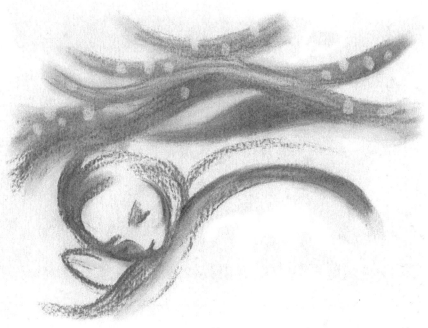

NINE:
DREAMING CYCLES

The dream jolted me upright. I was not sure which was the reality, me in my nightgown rubbing my eyes, or me walking on a trail in the brilliant sunlight. It was startling. I was in my private space, allowing my own experiment with sacred retreat during Nature's gift: the dream was a complete surprise.

I dreamed I was walking down a trail in the woods when I encountered a bear and a mountain lion. While I had dreamed of each animal separately in the past, I had never encountered both of them in a single dream. Additionally, each time I had previously dreamed of either, it had been very clear to me that they had come in my dream to help me. *This* time I was terrified. They approached me and began to rip the flesh off my bones. They persisted until I was completely consumed, and then they spit me out in a new form.

My dream terror vanished, for in the dream, I myself

disappeared until my dream animals gave me new life. With the new arrangement of my bones in the shiny new skin of my dream body, I proceeded down the trail until I came to a hidden waterfall. I approached it, stretching out my hand to touch the shimmering, azure water. In the dream, I noticed my hand and the water were the same: transparent, sparkling, and beautiful. I was connected to water. I awakened from that dream a different person.

It took days for the magnitude of that dream to sink in. I knew things about the world that I didn't know before. I understood that I was a divine part of Nature; I was connected to everything much more deeply than my preconceived mental concepts of relationship. My heart was full of compassion.

I gradually realized I had experienced a shamanic dream that broke me apart and put me back together in a more whole and holy way. The dream and the spirit animals that came to help appeared in the time and place I had set aside as sacred for my ceremony of cleansing and renewal during Nature's gift. They certainly cleaned me up and renewed who I was! From this dream, I now completely understood the sanctity of the Nature's gift in my own life, and I wanted to share it with other women. I knew it was important to withdraw into ourselves to purge, receive, and create, and that dreaming was part of the process.

While I have always been a vivid dreamer, in the past my dreams had been unpredictable. Sometimes they were the confused dreams that processed my day or worked out some troubling issue I was struggling with. Sometimes they were prescient dreams, informing me of possible danger. But I never knew what type of dream would arrive in the night. This dream had come at a specific phase of my bleeding cycle during a particular time when I was seeking growth and understanding.

I had recorded my dreams for some time, and now I decided to note the time of the month each dream occurred. I noticed with great interest that the deeply insightful dreams *only* occurred if I allowed the time and space for guidance by sleeping alone in my sacred space, and they were also more frequent during the time of Nature's gift. Apparently what my Blackfoot friend had told me was absolutely valid. Sleeping alone to quest for insight during my own cycle had brought me a vision and a new understanding of how to approach my life.

Researchers have classically defined dreams as symbols, images, sounds, sights, smells, tastes, and motor activities that occur during sleep to process daily experiences. People vary a lot in their need for sleep. Some dream researchers have suggested that when a portion of oneself is not integrated into awareness, more time must be spent in dealing with it separately in the dream state. According to this view, it could be implied that dreaming helps integrate a person's awareness and spiritual dream experiences could enhance that integration. Shamanic understanding extends the definition to include the wisdom of non-ordinary reality that arrives when our ordinary consciousness has been laid to rest. Shamanic dreams come more readily if we prepare for them and create a sacred space for the dream guides to visit.

In a cross-cultural comparison of dreaming among sixteen Native American tribes, Krippner and Thompson determined that each of the investigated cultures placed key values on dreams. In most of the Native American models, it was found that "the dream often represents the dreamer's merging with the 'unknown' visionary realm which can enlighten and empower the dreamer...the spirit world is the source of dreams" (18). Jeanne Achterberg takes a similar stance about allowing boundaries to merge in order to receive guidance saying,

"The mystic experience that brings knowledge and insight from sources beyond, can only happen if the barriers separating self from nonself become fluid, and the imagination reaches out beyond the intellect" (19). The prevalent North American indigenous beliefs about dreams as discovered in the Krippner-Thompson study could be summarized as follows

- Blackfoot--It is believed that dreams are produced by dream spirits who manifest in dreams as messengers, often in animal form. These dream spirits appear to bestow valuable gifts or information;
- Crow--Dreams come from the spirit world. The dreamer is in communication with the spirit world;

- Kwakiutl--Dreams represent direct contact with spiritual realms;
- Maricopa--Spiritual power comes only in dreams;
- Mojave--Dreams are the link between human beings and the spiritual world;
- Objibwa--All knowledge is the result of dreams.

Among Australian Aboriginals, blood imagery provides a link between dreaming and the perceivable world. The body needs the nourishing energy of the blood to maintain itself, and the blood purportedly needs "subtle energies" from the spirit world, which is attained through dreams. Recognizing the dream connection between energy from the spirit world and the physical body's energy maintains communication between them. Based on this indigenous view of the connection between blood and dreaming and the indigenous practice of separation during menses, one could conclude that the content of dream guidance during a particular time of month is a valuable asset.

It has been shown that women have more vivid and more meaningful dreams during their menstrual cycle. My original study yielded important insights about when and how women can most easily receive dream guidance. Dreams during menses may be more useful to women and to their communities, because women can receive more inspiration, illumination, creative ideas, or spiritual guidance during this time, if they have a private, sacred space for dreaming.

As already mentioned, there is a relationship between the level of estrogen in a woman's body and her frequency of dreaming, as well as her dream recall. Dream images are often vivid and understanding of dreams is typically guided by the emotion experienced in the dream. Women are more closely connected to their emotional state during the luteal phase of their cycle, and they dream more dreams that they designate as "important" during this phase. Yet there is no guidepost in our culture to instruct a woman to connect the dots between being emotional labile and dream wisdom. There is no map that shows us how to invite the dream and then follow the emotional trail it leaves for guidance.

I believe the first step to understanding the importance of our dreaming is to accept the validity of our emotional experience. I suggest we explore this more deeply, for understanding the cyclical timing of women's dreams could lead to important discoveries for all human dreaming. We need to learn that if we are upset by a dream, it has something instructive to tell us; the dream is telling us to make a change. If we are happy from a dream, we can surmise that we are being encouraged to move in *that* direction.

Not only do we need to stop chalking up the surge of premenstrual emotions to a chemical (only) change, we also need to start accepting the emotional cues of our dreams as guidelines. Emotional signs are pretty clear: a negative emotion indicates we should move away from a situation; a positive emotion encourages us to continue in a particular direction. If we learn to listen to our dreams from an emotional standpoint, we can garner much information to effectively guide us everyday. Withdrawing into a private retreat space as our hormones are preparing the way for the emotional map and the dream pointers only makes sense.

Most dreamers are aware of the transcendent quality of Shamanic dreams or guidance dreams. These dreams represent a different reality from ordinary reality, bringing the dreamer into a more revered place where spiritual guidance is more meaningful. Some dreams seem to be actual experiences, and if one accepts the premise that both waking and sleeping experiences are authentic, we find that is true. If real experiences elicit feelings and guide one's actions, which I believe they do, transcendent dreaming experiences are as real as our everyday reality. We simply don't share that reality with others in the same way we participate in the consensual reality of everyday life. To a dreamer, dreams can help shape the way she views the world. If we can follow the symbols of dreams and glean their meaning, dreams can make as much if not more sense than our waking experience.

If one takes the approach that dreams mirror insight and personal growth, paying attention to one's dreams is exceptionally important. Dreams mark changes in one's life and serve as guidelines for changes that need to occur. Respecting dream guidance by inviting the dream guides into a sacred space during a time of quest (vision quest for men or menstrual retreat questing for women) could be one of the most important elements for personal growth and spiritual understanding. Dreams are special messages that have meaning to the dreamer. No dream can be fully interpreted without the participation of the dreamer, for only she knows the feeling state of the dream. If we don't treat our dreams with respect by trying to remember and act upon their guidance, their importance and their impact are wasted. We move through our lives doing the motions of living without understanding the meaning of the choices we make. If we honor our dreams and incorporate the spiritual meaning that is offered at the right time and in the right place, our lives can be greatly enhanced.

Many spiritual traditions teach that the reality we accept as the truth is only a dream of a higher reality. I believe we are in a waking dream in our ordinary living. We are the co-creators of consensus reality through our waking dreams. Einstein taught us that all material things come from energy and quantum physics confirms this truth. Energy produces our thoughts and our dreams. Dreaming produces the guidance and the map to follow in our daily life. If we want to improve our lives and bring healing to our world, listening to our dreams in our waking life is paramount. We enlarge our dream guidance by adhering to a retreat time where we can invite our dreams to guide us during the biological time of our cycles when we are more *available* to listening.

We have more power to co-create than we realize. We must acknowledge that our biological time of retreat enables us to be more emotionally open to receive dream guidance that may be used to co-create our reality. If we honor our cycles and retreat to listen during Nature's gift, we receive the guidance we need to correct things that are unbalanced in our lives, to create solutions to challenges, and to bring greater harmony into our families and our world. The relationship between dreaming in a separate, sacred space during Nature's gift and the wisdom we receive is enormous. The dream space is very personal territory, and I encourage you to invite your own dream guides to visit. Create the time and space, and make them welcome. The power of our dreams can change our lives.

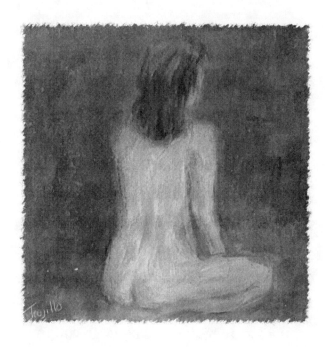

LIFE GIVER
—*Rebecca Smith Orleane*

As a woman life giver
Let me give birth
To each new moment
From joyful divinity within me

Remembering
To love myself, my neighbors, and my enemies,
For surely we are
Connected as One.

TEN:
CREATIVITY CYCLES

Wouldn't it be wonderful if everyone recognized our possibilities for creativity and regeneration? For women there is a biological four-step process that applies to creating new life or new ideas: purify, listen and incubate, create, bloom. We know this process in relationship to creating a child. The body needs to be purified, cleansed of all the "junk" to make a healthier home for the child we are to carry. The special state of incubation called pregnancy allows the seed to germinate, to whisper to us in the dark from our wombs, to kick and move as we feel the new life beginning to grow. The magical moment of seeing our creation arrives through the birth process. The creative process continues daily, as we watch the being we have given life bloom and grow, hopefully, into a member of the human species that contributes to life on our planet. This creative process may be used by women to create new life or to create new ideas, projects, and circumstances. The same creative process is available for men as well; only men are lacking the biological guidance to help them understand the importance of honoring cycles of creativity.

We can apply the above formula to creatively bringing forth anything in our lives. Because of our biology, women are the models for creation in the human species, yet our culture treats the creative process lightly if it doesn't involve an acclaimed work of art or a live birth. Daily living involves creativity, yet daily living is rarely referred to as "art." I believe that's wrong: there is an art to living that involves some stage of creativity every moment. We should be aware that we are birthing our lives through our attitudes and our actions, and it is through understanding the process deeply that we can make lasting change.

For years psychologists have studied creativity. Krippner defined creativity as any act, idea, or product that creates changes in an existing domain, or that transforms parts of an existing domain into a new one. Anderson defined creativity as the ability to deal adequately and originally with a new situation or to deal innovatively with an old one. Russ said that creativity encompasses divergent and fluid thinking, free association, and transformation abilities. May said true creators are those who give birth to some new reality. Emilie Conrad provided my favorite definition of creativity saying, "It is the emerging unexpected, the opposite of control and predictability. The creative consciousness is always listening in between; it is not a focused awareness, it is an omni-directional awareness" (20). None of these definitions support the idea that creativity is the exclusive domain of specially, gifted artists. These definitions tell us that creativity is something we are all capable of. In fact, as I will explain, it is our divine right and is necessary for life.

The wonderful work of creativity maven Dr. Ruth Richards has shown us that we are all creative and that creativity does not exist only in moments of artistic genius. She has defined creativity as doing something new in the course of one's activity at work or at leisure. Richards has suggested that we must first embrace ourselves in order to embrace the kind of creativity that provides ultimate uniqueness along with ultimate interconnectedness (21). The focus of Richards' work is to teach us to value creativity as part of everyday life. Richards tells us that everyday creativity should not be seen as a new idea, for it is a fundamental survival capability. The ability to be creative is a key aspect of mental health and is a core property of all living beings. Ruth Richards has listed seven important points to consider about the necessity of creativity in our lives. I can add to these reasons, but I cannot improve upon what she has said, and the merit of her understanding bears listing these seven points here as we recreate our myths. Creativity:

1- is not an optional "extra" for all but certain famous

people, but rather, is an essential capability for survival and ongoing development.

2- is not limited to special areas such as the arts, but, rather, it can be found in all parts of life.

3- is not merely a light and pleasant diversion, but, rather, is a vital enterprise involving deep commitment, concentration, risk taking, and sometimes-personal transformation.

4- although sometimes unsettling, it is not fundamentally an enterprise that unsettles and evokes pathology, but rather, is one that can open, integrate, and heal.

5- is not an endeavor focused only on end products, but rather involves a healthy way of approaching life, which connects us more meaningfully to our world, whether we are actively creating or appreciating the creativity of others.

6- is not an activity set apart from much of our being, but rather is one that reaches deep into mind, body, and spirit, and can help heal us, revealing a profound mind-body-connection we are only beginning to understand.

7- is not a neutral or safe activity, that risks little, but, rather, can be a potentially dangerous enterprise offering disruption and change- including personal reorganization, and potential threats to society's status quo. Against these forces of change may be arrayed powerful obstacles, internal, and external, conscious and unconscious. But we cannot address them unless we know why our creativity may be eclipsed and "hidden" to begin with" (22).

I believe creativity is born from either a place of joy that wants to add beauty and harmony to life, or from a place of inward discontent that knows change is necessary, or possibly both. But whatever is happening whenever a person moves towards creativity, they are involved in listening. Without listening to what needs to change or to what is asking to be created, creativity does not happen. Creativity is intimately linked to listening to the divine whisper of something larger than us, something that plants the idea within us and guides our thoughts and actions to bring the idea into reality.

Creation requires connection with divinity, and divinity is connected to beauty and joy. A person involved with creating beauty feels joy, a feeling connected with higher consciousness and the experience of honoring one's own potential. In other words, *each* of us holds the potential to be creative on a daily basis and, to thereby heighten our own moods and improve our own lives. There is joy in any creation, I believe, because it either adds something to the world or it relieves us from an intolerable place of stagnation. Without creativity in our lives, we become increasingly depressed, or we simply die.

One reason so many people disallow their own creativity

is that they are uncomfortable claiming their own divinity. The two go together. To create is divine; to be divine allows creation. Unfortunately, Christianity has taught that only God is "the creator" and only *that* divinity can create. We have disassociated ourselves from understanding that we are all divine and we all have the ability to be creative. Women manifest the gift of creation through every pregnancy and birth. Yet many of us have dismissed the little creations we accomplish on a daily basis, dismissing them as unimportant or dismissing them from fearful thinking that we might be claiming some of God's territory if we call ourselves creators. We cannot blasphemously take the place of God, for we *are* part of the divine: we were intended to be co-creators when we were given the opportunity to listen and the capacity to think. The path to creativity is to listen, to think, to act.

If we have trouble believing that we are part of a larger divinity, we will also have trouble believing that we have the power to create, or that what we do is creative. Swallowing Christian humility out of fear of blasphemy that we, too, are creators, or accepting a smaller vision of ourselves, does not allow us to *be* the powerful co-creators that we actually are. Further, we give away our power when we do not accept our divine ability to create and when we claim that only someone smarter and more talented, or something greater than ourselves can create. We are connected to that larger source and, when we allow it, it will show us the what and how and when of every creative moment, reminding us that *every* moment has the potential to be a creative one.

Although the definition of creative persons in most cultures includes such personality traits as risk-taking and openness, I believe creativity is a process available to all people at some level in everyday life. Creativity enjoys a certain freedom that allows for listening to guidance and inspiration; it involves a willingness to let go of being governed by the usual standards for thought and action. A meal created for one's family can be more creative than a piece of art if it is innovative, beautiful, and outside the expected norm. And certainly a newfound solution to a long-standing relationship problem is creatively valuable, for such a creative gift can bring more harmony into everyday living. Everyday creativity is our birthright and offers the way to make a world of beauty and harmony. The more we accept that we *can* make changes, the more we listen to what needs to change; the more we act on inspiration we receive, the more we honor who we are as spiritual humans.

Remember my list of stages of creativity: purification, listening and incubation, creation, blooming. From the point of view of women's cycles, preparation for creativity involves cleansing out what is no longer needed and making space. Whether it is the nine months required to incubate a child before it is brought into the light of the world, or quiet time to incubate a new idea or project, the quiet reverie of a retreat during Nature's gift allows an opportunity for cleaning out the old, listening, intuiting and, finally incubating what is to come next. The retreat where one is withdrawn from daily affairs allows for the incubation that is part of the process. The incubation time is the place of deep listening, the place where divine inspiration can be seeded into our consciousness. While it sometimes may seem that we spontaneously arrive at a new solution or a new idea, if we have not honored the cycle of resting and listening, the time of incubation, there would have been no energy or space for the new idea to arrive. Richards points out that creativity involves being spontaneous, free, open to experience, able to live more vividly in the moment (as opposed to the past or future), being resilient when shaken up, being consciously aware, listening to a higher calling, and being appreciative of our fundamental interdependence, as well as the effect we have on each other and the world. She suggests that we should consider creativity as involving the give and take of all that we routinely experience from each other and our surroundings and as important to us as the air, water, food, and other resources we take in. Ruth Richards boldly states, "When I hear another person speak, my brain is altered- accessing memories, sending new chemical signals, likely growing new dendrites" (23). Because of the power of our natural interconnection, we should *always* be aware of and responsible for how we affect others in the environment around us.

Many researchers connect illumination experiences, or

being able to experience things in a new creative way to the body more than to cognitive awareness. The body seems to convey understanding of new experiences to the mind, where cognitive translation puts the experiences into words for communication to others. Yet it is the body that actually records and reflects the change and acts on the inspiration, either through heightened brain chemistry or the actual creation that is born from the inner understanding.

This is not necessarily a new idea. The Kolish Indians believed illumination stemmed from the body awareness a young girl obtained during her first menses. The blood-transformation changes women experience give them a bodily knowledge of their own creativity. This perspective lends credence to the notion that women understand the creative process through their own body awareness, and can teach others by example how to honor creative cycles. It is through our allowing space and time for deep listening in harmony with the timing our bodies dictate, that creative guidance occurs. This phenomenon has its roots in psychobiological development.

Menstruation is the first timing secret related to blood for women, and pregnancy is the second. Both are related to creativity. Both pregnancy and menstrual bleeding are related to the incubation stage of creativity; when we allow ourselves to listen from the quiet of a sacred space during these times, creative illumination blossoms and are often followed by a creative product, whether that is a child, a work of art, or a new idea. Understanding and allowing this process helps us manifest more ideas, greater problem solving, or new thoughts, as well as helping us to take the initiative to produce new products or to finish old ones.

Myths from many indigenous societies tell of beliefs that menstruation is a powerful time for change and creativity. One of the foremost scholars of cultural myths, Joseph Campbell, pointed out that one function of myths is to put one's way of life in accord with Nature. Perhaps women's biological urge to slow down and be quiet during the time they are losing blood is a form of balancing one's life with Nature. I am certainly an advocate of this point of view. Indigenous people around the world have encouraged women to retire from everyday duties during Nature's gift as the way to bring fresh ideas back to their communities. If one purpose of myths is to help humans align with Nature, to see the harmony and beauty of that alignment, and explain how others have made the journey, the return of treating of Nature's gift as a sacred reality with the power to open our own creativity is quite valuable. Rollo May pointed out three decades ago that we should be able to retire from a world that is too much with us and be quiet to let the solitude work for us and through us. Women's natural biological cycle is a key for all humans to listen to the timing of our own bodies and to accept the creative spark of life, both within us and flowing towards us. Acknowledging our own creativity and our own divine spark keeps us alive. Remember, life is change. Change is *always* involved in creativity. If we allow ourselves to be non-changing, we die. Cardiologist Ary Goldberger noted,

"The healthy heartbeat is not regular and rhythmic, but contains chaotic irregularities that actually determine the organ's health and the individual's survival." (24)

Ruth Richards points out the significance that our brains react the same whether we imagine something or actually encounter it.

Women have always had a special time Nature sets aside for us to expel the old and make room for the new. We need to learn to *use* it properly. Down gear, empty, expel what is not needed. Cleanse, ask for guidance, listen, and *wait*. The inspiration will come just from *being* during this important time. It is not the time to "do". The doing will be accomplished more efficiently and quicker when the time and space to receive guidance and conceive creative ideas has been respected. If we honor our own natural timing and model our respect of cycles for others, everyone will benefit from understanding the value of slowing down, listening, and accepting creativity as part of our divine nature.

While hundreds of researchers have looked at what causes eminent creativity (the kind that produces extraordinary pieces of art or brilliant ideas) and everyday creativity (the kind I have been talking about in this chapter), it is apparent to me that one of the greatest downsides of our patriarchal culture is that it has cut us off from our sense of connection to Nature, to our own divinity, and to our own innate creativity. Examining what causes people to be creative does not look at what is missing when people are not creative. What I am about to say may be seen by some as radical, but it is true. When Christian patriarchal culture changed the structure of our belief systems and our myths, we lost much of our potential to be fully human. When women's cycles were dismissed, dishonored, and disempowered, what women have to teach about cycling through life in accord with Nature was silenced.

The male model for progressive thinking and action has squeezed us into a too tight place of living, one that is hurried and harried, where we perceive that we "do not have time" to slow down to smell the roses, to listen to the still small voice of our intuition or our spiritual guidance, or to connect with another life in a meaningful way, at least for any length of time. Human connection has been downsized to a quick sexual encounter or to stealing an afternoon for lunch with a friend. Even our seeking exercise, which can be a wonderful way of connecting with Nature, is often confined to a brief visit to the gym.

Linear progressive thought and a value system that focuses on constant achievement and advancement has left little time for listening to our inner guidance. Our creativity has been dashed through the pressure of crunching time to get more done. Our creativity has been shut down by our belief that there is only one creator (God as Creator) who endowed only certain "special" individuals to create. We are not aware that we have the God-given ability ourselves to create in our more ordinary lives. We need to begin to connect the dots between our divinity and our everyday creative abilities.

Lastly, our creativity has been limited because of our separation from Nature and our egotistic self-centeredness as humans. We are *not* the best of God's creations, nor are we necessarily highest on the chain of intellect, compassion, or interest in our environment. (Look at those attributes in dolphins and whales to see how we are lacking.) We are, perhaps, the species with the largest ego and the greatest desire to control others. Humanity seems to be moving more and more into the direction of separating ourselves from the rest of Nature. Technological advances speed us up and simultaneously reinforce the values that will ultimately destroy us. The more we move away from being part of Nature and honoring our living cycles (especially women's bleeding cycles), the more we move towards death. Life is creativity. Life is change. We move towards death when we use our lives as a daily grind to "get things done", following the model for faster and faster progress. As Mahatma Gandhi said, "There is more to life than increasing its speed."

We must slow down. We must learn to listen. We must

make space for divine inspiration and intuition to guide us. We must create to be fully alive. We must honor our biological nature, and we must come back to recognizing that we are *part* of Nature, *not* her governors. Please, readers, consider what I am saying. Please allow time to really absorb the possibilities of being in the world in another way. *Can* you slow down? *Can* you change your values to allow time to listen? *Can* you accept that you are a divine part of Nature? *Can* you create through your thoughts, your ideas, your spontaneous insights and your intuition? The answers to how we live our lives are held in the slowness. As I move slower and slower, creating space, the creaking and popping I hear in my body reflects the dropping away of patterns and structures of who I am and how I am in the world. Silence, slow, moving waves, ripples of newness and possibility as I ride the wave of myself.

As I have discovered the gift of slowness for myself, I am making a plea to all who are reading this: *PLEASE STOP THE FAST PACE AND SLOW DOWN. PLEASE WORK ON UNDERSTANDING THAT YOU ARE DIVINE. PLEASE LISTEN TO THE CALL OF CREATIVITY AND INVITE HER IN. THE FEMININE PRINCIPLES OF LIFE ARE RETURNING; THEY ARE CALLING TO YOU!*

MY RIVER
—Rebecca Smith Orleane

My river lies in the

    Contours of my body-

        Like a river of Earth,

           She swells to the tides of passion

           And outflows her banks,

              Laying fertile grounds

                For seeds of new growth.

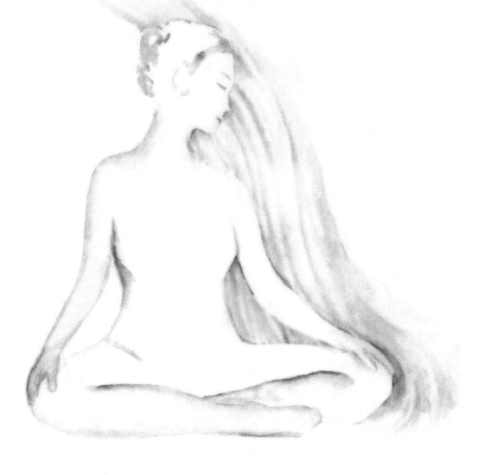

ELEVEN:
WOMEN AND WATER

A woman's heart moves like water, flowing and responding to each motion it encounters. Like a pebble tossed into a still, quiet lake, ripples of love travel from a single small touch, flowing outwards until the effects are felt on the farthest shore. Likewise, when a woman cries, anyone around can feel the ripples of sadness emanating from her heart.

How are women like water? Let's start by looking at the connection between water and life. Science has proven that life originated in the sea. Science has also shown the chemical similarities between ocean water and blood, both made of salt and water. The human fetus is surrounded by sea-like amniotic fluid. As an embryo, humans are 97% water; at birth, our water element can be measured at 78%; by adulthood, our body water rangers from 52% to 70%, with women traditionally having more water than men. Marks, author of <u>The Holy Order of Water</u>, encapsulates the importance of water saying,

"If life did begin with the sea, then we are alive only because we carry the sea within us" (25). We are made of water, and understanding that makeup helps us to relate to life with a greater sense of flow. Water, in its liquid state, always flows. Robert Gardner distinguishes the exact parameters of water in the human body, saying,

"Of the 52 - 70% water in our bodies, 60% of that lies within the living cells, and another 25% is found between cells. The brain is 85% water. Blood plasma holds 8%, and 5% acts either as a lubricant for joints or fills cavities of organs such as our eyes. Blood is 90% water; kidney tissue is 8% water; our muscles are 75% water; the liver is 66% water; and even "dry" bone is 33% water. We drink about 6,600 gallons of water in a lifetime and about five times our body weight each year (26).

Gardner's "dry" (pun intended) statistics give a factual representation of just how important water is to human life. Expanding the statistical makeup of our human bodies to a "wetter, juicier" more lyrical feminine understanding of human connection to water, offers a deeper respect for the wetness of life. Water sustains us, and allows us to flow through biological and emotional changes. Women's biological makeup commands a higher percentage of water, and it flows out of us in the form of our blood. The wet blood of our bodies is the moisture that brings forth life. From this bodily understanding, we may hold a greater respect for the link between water and life

In looking at the myths of an earlier time, there are many references to the connections between women and water. Water has been referred to as the blood of the earth. In Mesopotamia, streams and caves, the source of rivers, were likened to the vagina of the earth. Indeed, in Babylonia, the term pu meant both *source of a river* and *vagina*. Samaria also used the same word (buru) for *vagina* and for *river*. Actually, women are like water in many ways. Author Theodore Schwenk has eloquently expressed specific qualities held by water (or life; Schwenk interchanges the words emphasizing the connection.) I quote him here, using artistic license to interchange the words *water* and *life* with *woman, adding* parenthetical comments. Notice the similarities in the attributes Schwenk gives to water/life and the attributes that are so large a part of the feminine way of being.

"Life *(woman)* works chiefly as a synthesizer, forming wholes that are greater than the sum of all their parts. *(Women balance many small things, different parts of life, in order to have a better-ordered total).* Life *(woman)* moves rhythmically, not, however, in a mechanically measured beat. Life *(woman)* is always a little bit eccentric. Life *(woman)* is responsive to cosmic rhythms, indeed, entirely governed by them *(woman's cycles).* Therefore, it *(she)* flows with the flow of time, in cycles rather than in straight-line or a mechanical hook up *(needing to follow her body's timing rather than a calendar.)* Life *(woman)* always leaves itself *(herself)* free space for maneuvering *(nothing is definite because change is always possible);* it *(she)* never submits to exact calculation *(reserving the right to change her mind.)* It *(she)* moves in cycles wherein metamorphoses and heightenings take place. It *(she)* is attuned to the cosmos *(life's rhythms and her rhythms)* and to endlessness in time and space *(ever noticed that mothers have a reputation for being able to be everywhere and see everything at once?)* In every area water *(woman)* assumes the role of mediator (27) *(how many women are the peacemakers in their families or in the workplace?)*

This poetic license with Schwenk's valuable work is by no means intended to demean the worth of his observations. It's just that in reading his work, I kept noting the similarities between the feminine way of consciousness and the water of life.

I asked a man whose opinion I deeply value how he sees women being like water? He responded that women, like water, start to go one way and then they go another quite unpredictably. I think, for the more linear, constant gender, this quality must, at times, be quite exasperating. As women, it is our responsibility to show men the many benefits of our cyclic, sometimes unpredictable nature and help them navigate our changeability with more ease.

When I think of the many qualities of water, I am amazed at how often women approximate those qualities as we navigate our lives. Our language is full of colorful phrases demonstrating camaraderie between women and water. Consider such water based phraseology as: *"She flowed from one task to another;"* or *"Her heart melted;"* or" *She was wet with excitement;"* or *"Her heart was cold as ice;"* or *"She was so angry you could see steam coming from her ears!"* Each of these comparisons invokes water qualities (ice, steam, or melting liquid) to express an attribute of a woman's experience.

Women are like water in their problem solving abilities, although we may or may not be aware of just how powerful we are in the ways we meet obstacles. Think of a stream flowing calmly through the land. When a river or stream finds a rock in its path, there are several ways the stream can proceed without having its journey blocked or deterred. The water can gently splash against the rock until continued exposure erodes the rock, or it can easily move around the rock, finding another path, unimpeded. The rock might stay firm in its place, or it might come loose from the water's gentle movement and begin to travel in the same direction. These water-like movements are familiar to women as tools for handling difficult situations. We are much like rivers and streams in our fluid negotiation of life.

When confronted with a seemingly insurmountable obstacles (like the rock in the stream), using the feminine quality leads to more gentle solutions. Most women are naturally peacemakers, striving to find peaceful or cooperative solutions to daily obstacles. Using male tactics (trying to be like men rather than honoring our native feminine aspects) can cause women to appear pushy, aggressive, and hostile in interactions. When we use our feminine nature, most women, like water, are far more likely to choose to flow around an obstacle or gently reintroduce a point, rather than to use a more forceful tactic. We understand gentle persistence when something is blocking our path. We also know the incredible power of simply flowing around an obstacle, allowing it to be what it is, while we continue on our own journey. Women also know there is greater force in making peaceful changes that allows others to choose their own paths.

While women naturally reflect the power of the feminine in their being, it is important to acknowledge that women do not *own* feminine principles. There is a feminine part to all of us, and men who connect to the feminine qualities within themselves are much more balanced and effective in living. I am troubled by the fact that many women have adopted masculine models for dealing with conflict, rather than using their more powerful feminine abilities. Women in our culture have become separated from realization that feminine power can be greater than forceful, masculine power, because our culture devalues feminine attributes systemically. It is a tragedy to see women model themselves after the gender than has ignored them, emulating the principles that have caused the suppression of feminine values. It is imperative that we remember that feminine qualities support life. We must stop copying men, fighting to achieve what we want, and move back towards our innate peaceful navigation of life, inviting men to join us in using the power of the feminine.

In our peacemaking roles, women attempt to join what is divided and unite it again with the whole. The feminine principle asks us to continually remember that we are one, and to join each other in harmony. Women have an advantage in peacemaking endeavors, for we are whole-brain thinkers; we use our entire brain, joining right-brained creative thinking through the corpus collusum to our left brained analytical thinking.

One place we can see the presence of peaceful joining and water is looking at ceremonies throughout the world. Christian baptisms use sprinkling of or emersion in water to celebrate the "birth" of the new Christian soul. The Jewish faith observes ritual *mikvah* baths, through which the water changes spiritual status and acts as purification. Native Americans connect to spiritual guidance through River Plunges and Sweat Lodges. In each of these traditions, the person emerges purified, changed, and with a "clean start or *a new life*." The connection here to water and women is simple: each of these ceremonies uses water as a symbol of life *(life is not possible without passing through the water-blood of a woman.)* Women carry the most celebrated ceremony within our own bodies: the ritual of monthly bleeding (which *should* be treated as a holy ceremony) announces the possibility of bringing forth new life.

The deep wisdom held in each woman's body connects water and life and death. Every month, women have the opportunity to bring forth life or to dispel the blood that life would have been. There is connection. Every woman's cycle holds death and life in perfect balance, as the blood that is not needed for a new baby is sloughed off, along with the opportunity to slough off everything else that has not been working in a woman's life. Worldwide, women have deeply understood the connections of water to life and death.

Ethnographic studies have shown that many indigenous cultures throughout the world have compared the life-giving blood of women to the life-giving water of Mother Earth. Blood contains life and stands for life itself. Historically menstruation was believed to evoke a feminine power more potent than any power a man could have. Men have often feared that they would be "overpowered by this most potent of sacred substances, a holy fluid specific to females" (28).

The blood of our Earth (our rivers and our streams) and the blood of women have today lost their ceremonial value. There is a similarity in the disrespect our culture has shown to both water and women. Both have been used as a commodity, polluted with disregard, blocked or dammed to prevent the natural flow of change that both water and women bring. The emotional waters of women crying for necessary changes have been dammed and damned.

Emotions are related to water because they are fluid and changeable. Like water, emotions can nourish us or, if blocked, or if too fierce, they can harm us and those around us. Knowing how to listen to rising emotions in a timely manner is no different than knowing how to interact with the ocean's tides. Water and women are both affected by gravitational pulls of the moon, and both respond to the pull of the tides. This tidal pull governs our menstrual cycles and holds sway over our emotions, granting us the great gift of emotional expression. Culturally women's emotional volatility has often been spurned as detrimental, however I believe it is through unblocked, unrepressed, free flow of feeling that a woman meets her challenges and navigates the changes necessary in her life. The emotions of anger, grief, and compassion guide us in the directions we need to travel. When the waters of emotion swell for recognition and we do not allow them to flow, we often choose the wrong path. Continued repression of the waters of emotions is no different than blocking of a river. Eventually the river will overflow its banks, and the flood can be devastating.

Let me make it clear that I am not a fan of histrionic expression of emotion. I am not advocating that we should respond to every unsettling incident in our lives with an outburst of tears or a blast of angry words. I am proposing that through the sacred retreat process put forth in this book, women learn to *listen* to what their emotions are telling them and *act* on the guidance of their intuitive states. The gift of being in harmony with the tides of the ocean keeps us connected to Nature in ways that a man cannot be, and it is our responsibility to honor that connection through our daily living, modeling it for others.

I have moved through the waters of emotion in my own life, ebbing and flowing with the tears that moved me emotionally (and literally) from one place to another. When tears flow, there is movement, just as when a river flows there is movement. According to Cherokee tradition, it is a good practice to "go to the water" every day, at the beginning of the day and at the end of the day. Each time you ask the river to take from you what is not yours or what is not needed and to bring you what you do need. Hawk Littlejohn taught me that if you do not live near water or the water is frozen in winter, you do this practice mentally, imagining yourself dipping into the water with intention, asking for movement. The Cherokee call it plunging; a spiritual plunge is ritual immersion seven times, each time clearing you from what you do not need and bringing to you what you do need. I believe the Cherokee understood that we can blend our own human water to the waters of Mother Earth and learn how to be more fluid in our lives.

Living our cycles in a way that they spiral upward in growth is one way of doing that. We are not meant to live in a manner that pushes against our polar opposites, expressing the conflict of our duality. Rather we are meant to experience our cycles as a way of moving towards a wider array of possibilities and greater unity. Women have a greater understanding of connection and unity. Women need to honor our cycles to invite possibility and to help the world move towards unity. Cycles and movement bring possibility, understanding, resolution, and peace, peace, peace. It is unnatural for water to remain still. Water by its essential nature is always moving, and by constantly moving it serves to create, protect, energize, nourish, and sustain life. Women are like water, because we, like water, move towards creating conditions conducive to life.

Anishanabec people called women the keepers of the Water. As such, it was the responsibility of women to teach respect for the Spirit of Water, which gives life to everything else. Women as life givers, and water as life giver, shared a deep connection. It is natural that women understand the power of water as they feel its movement through them with monthly regularity. It also makes sense that since women understand the connection of water to bringing forth life, we have the responsibility to care for water. Caring for water goes beyond caring for water outside of us. If we are made of water, which certainly we are, we must care for our inner waters and the inner waters of others, for we are all drops of the same ocean. We are connected, and we need to recognize that, as water beings, we share a level of communication with every bit of water on the planet. This understanding can profoundly change our relationships. Caring for another's water is, quite simply, living in love.

In her pioneering book, Life on Land, Emilie Conrad addresses the connection of water to love. She writes,

"In an amazing way, water also brings us the quality of love- a love that is beyond human possession, beyond altruism, perhaps a love that we are yet to realize. The movement of fluid within us is characterized by wave motion. These undulating wave motions become increasingly more subtle as every part of us begins to shimmer with the memory of our origin. The caresses of these fluid waves bring about an erotic, sensual, spiritual union- a cosmic return that words cannot even begin to describe. Wave motions represent not only our biological rapport with the universe; they rock us in a lush cradle. It took me many years to recognize that the undulating fluid that I felt in my body is the movement of love. Looking back, it seems so obvious- that the undulating waves of primordial motion are the movements of love. Not emotional love, but an encompassing atmosphere of love. A love that has its own destiny. Perhaps using humans as its messengers, this love is trying to land on Earth" (29).

In his wonderful book The Holy Order of Water, William Marks speaks of romantic love, saying, "When two people fall in love, the water in every cell of their being resonates in harmony" (30). This cellular resonance is something a woman is familiar with in the biology of her cells, having felt it from the moon's pull on her internal waters from her first menstrual cycle. It is no surprise to experience cellular resonance of her body's waters when she moves into emotional connection with another human being, whether that is her lover or her child. When one is in perfect resonance with the right person, the astounding resonance is simultaneously exhilarating and familiar. You flow towards the other person because your water recognizes and knows the rightness of his water. I waited my whole life for my heartmate, who brought me instant understanding of this truth. When I first hugged my heartmate, I knew something was different and special about our connection. The water of my body stirred with a peaceful resonance. I believe that the water in his body was speaking to the water in my body, through the rhythmic beating of our hearts. While we were getting to know each other, we relied on written words, yet my body, remembering the rightness of the first hug, continued to send and receive messages through the water of my being to my heart and my brain. When I next heard his voice (which was some long time later), my heart burst forth in rainbow colors and flooded my whole body with love.

The resonance of love moves through us like water. We need to reinstate honor to both water and women, recognizing that all of life depends upon both. Women need to return to using feminine principles to guide their lives and to teach, by example that gentle motion can bring the necessary changes that guide us towards peace. Perhaps, through our very natures, we can bring the world more fluidity, harmony, and love. Our bodies hold wisdom and form. They are repositories of our experience, and how we move through our experiences dictates how we create our form. The menstrual cycle is a gate, allowing what needs to move in and out, appropriate to the connection of the flow. Our liquid crystalline bodies thrive on movement and flow. Like all bodies of water, we cleanse, change, and flow, allowing the rivers within us to moisten the land upon which we live. Healthy rivers, in us or on Earth, support life. We are connected to all through our water.

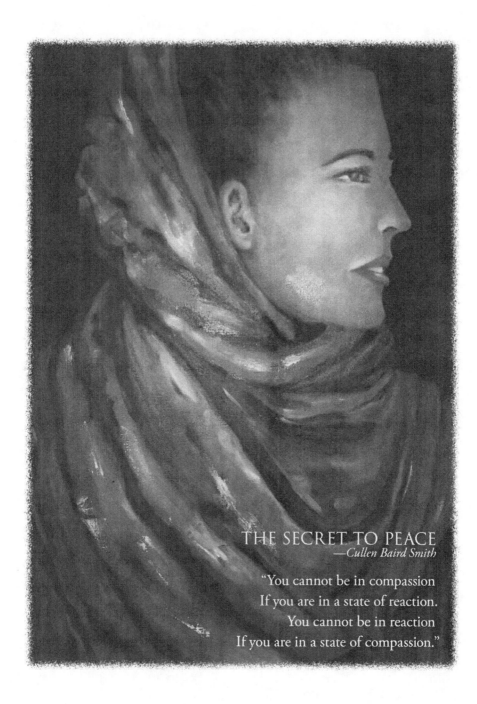

THE SECRET TO PEACE
—Cullen Baird Smith

"You cannot be in compassion
If you are in a state of reaction.
You cannot be in reaction
If you are in a state of compassion."

TWELVE:
MENOPAUSE MAGIC

The dual changing nature of being female brings a poignant understanding that life is not only full of change, but that life IS change. To live is to experience countless changes on a daily basis, and for women, for a large part of our lives even more changes occur within us once a month. Menopause moves us into another stage of change, a stage that is quite beautiful when we accept it as our coming into the full blossoming of being wise women, rather that lamenting it as the end of our youth. Christiane Northrup defines menopause as "an exciting developmental stage-one that, when participated in consciously, holds enormous promise for transforming and healing our bodies, minds, and spirits at the deepest levels" (31).

I believe that emotional problems many women have with menopause are culturally induced. To begin with, many of us have not honored our menstrual bleeding as a sacred time and allowed the cleansing and creative cycle. If we have not listened to and acted on the urgings for change that presented themselves throughout the life of our bleeding cycles, they build up until an untenable necessity for change comes screaming forth as we approach menopause. Suddenly, we are tired of putting everyone else first, and we are simply compelled to listen to and act upon the urgings coming forth like birth pains.

Dr. Christiane Northrup empowers our hormonal wisdom, saying, "Our hormones are giving us an opportunity to see, once and for all, what we need to change in order to live honestly, fully, joyfully, and healthfully in the second half of our lives" (32). I believe that the changes necessary for the second half of life come more gracefully and with less force if we have spent a lifetime of listening to those urgings every month as we bleed. If we have practiced listening and acting on the principal of change for our entire adult lives, it is easier to facilitate larger changes with grace and finesse. Purging what is not working, deeply listening for guidance, and creatively birthing new possibilities on a monthly basis in harmony with Nature paves the path to our wise-women years with ease rather than struggle.

An additional impediment to smooth menopause transition is our attachment to the Hollywood/Madison Avenue vision of a perfection that proclaims our value is attached to our youth. It is partially our own fault that such judgments land so hard when we reach menopause, for most of us have spent a lifetime accepting the cultural definition of beauty and worth. It upsets me no end when I see young women brandishing their breasts for show or hiding their natural beauty behind the latest brand of lipstick. While there is nothing wrong with enjoying our bodies and decorating them, the vision of our inner beauty has been lost to an external standard of what is required for acceptance and perfection.

Many women have been tricked into believing that they must stay young and productive forever in order to be loved. (Empty nest syndrome is a prime example of a women's struggle with feeling productive and needed. When the kids leave home, millions of women struggle to redefine their worth.) Worse, they fear that once they are no longer young and productive, they will be cast aside as useless. Menopause has even been defined as reaching the end of our "productive years." Because they are so deeply unaware of their value as creative beings, some women mourn the loss of being able to produce children, even if they have never *chosen* to give birth. They mourn the *opportunity* to bear a child. We must learn to deeply understand that creativity does not stop when we can no longer produce a child. I have sat with many of my clients as they bemoaned the approach of menopause for fear of being "tossed away." Only recently have menopausal women begun to understand and embrace the fact that the stage of menopause is a stage that not only holds wisdom, but can also be full of creativity and satisfaction. Our progressive patriarchal culture values improvement on the status quo, and it abhors unpredictability and change. Yet it is unpredictability and change that allow for creativity and that infuse us with life. Many of us have spent lifetimes defending, what seems to the more constant gender, unpredictable changes. How many times have you heard the confused, "But I thought you wanted...."? It is not men's fault that they are so easily confused by our changing states. *It is ours.* Very few of us have sat down and looked at or explained our dual way of being in the world, an existence that requires different things at different times. Instead, we have defended ourselves, offered surface explanations, and struggled to be more constant. By the time we reach menopause, most of us have felt the compelling pressure to at least *attempt* to stay static, or barring that, to hide the effects of our cyclical needs and make the best of the changes that occur. Changes that come in a woman's cycle are not linear, progressive, culturally sanctioned improvements. They are spiraling, creative, life affirming, and often surprisingly unpredictable.

While all menstruating women experience the biological phenomena of Menopause, it seems that only modern Western culture considers it a medical event. In this country, Menopause has been treated by many as a disease to be medicated, an abnormal imbalance. Like menstruation and the changes that occur premenstrually, menopause has been pathologized into something needing to medical attention. Fortunately, enlightened doctors like Dr. Christiane Northrup are spending a great deal of energy educating women about the gifts of Menopause and offering medical *support* as opposed to "medicating the problem away." After a lifetime of being belittled for being different, modern women are finally being educated by such gifted teachers as Dr. Northrup to see Menopause as an opportunity. I often refer to Menopause as the Second Coming of Women's Liberation.

To reiterate, I believe Menopause hits us hard in this culture for two reasons. The first has to do with our attitudes towards beauty, health, youth, and self esteem. The second reason Menopause affects women so severely in this culture is that many of us have lived a lifetime of not honoring the processes of being a woman, disconnected from our cyclical nature, hiding it, neither sharing our experiences nor using them to further our growth.

Many of us grew up in a time when it was not "politically correct" to be different once a month. Working mothers and career women, competing with men to be seen as equal did not know how to value our differences while climbing the corporate ladder, or we were just plain too busy and tired to take time for ourselves. Not only did we try to hide our cyclical nature, we were encouraged to do so everywhere we turned. Magazines, television, and employers who wanted maximum productivity told us "now you can be the same every day of the month!" The fact is, however, we have not been given permission or blessings to do what is *natural*, which is to be *different* during the month---to honor being receptive as equally important as being productive. Corporate business does not recognize the cycles of Nature that affect daily work rhythms. Neither do well-meaning spouses and partners who have come to seek constancy in relationships rather than being intrigued by the play of quiet and laughter, tears and joy, cleansing and creating. Until recently, very few women in our society were taught to value the natural time we have been given to clean out what isn't working, listen for guidance on what will work better, dream our dreams for a better life, incubate new ideas, then bring them into full bloom for family and society.

So just as we get accustomed to our monthly changes, whether we ignored them or whether we heralded them as the sacred times that they were, suddenly they are over. Or maybe not so suddenly- maybe Menopause creeps up on us, making us question who we are, as our bodies move into unfamiliar territory and our emotions come to the surface, like a top that has been wound too tight and suddenly let go. We start to miss a few periods, or they get a little lighter. Or they come more frequently and surprise us with their intensity. There is a huge surge reminding us of what it is to be a woman.

We may be afraid something is "wrong", but actually, this is the way it is meant to be. It is *different*, not *wrong*.

There may be an increase in tears or anger. Everything seems so intense. Things seems to matter in a way that has never been so important. Our partners, children, friends may look at us differently, as if we are different people, asking where has the woman gone who was so calm and predictable? They may question *who is* this person who is so angry, so weepy, so volatile in her moods? Why does she no longer want to do all the things she used to do, and why do things upset her that never did before?

I'm a "jump in feet first" kind of girl. I've lived most of my life jumping in feet first, taking on projects by "pulling everything out into the floor" (as my mother would refer to my childhood pattern of cleaning my closet), basically doing everything in a big way and all at once. When I started knitting, the first project I chose was a complicated sweater. I tend to jump in feet first with any idea or project that excites me; in fact, I cannot recall ever tackling a new project that I didn't try to learn everything about it all at once. Ironically, my body apparently understood this chosen pattern, because I also "jumped" into Menopause. There were no telltale signs sneaking up on me. I was just *there*. I went from regular monthly cycles to a complete cessation of bleeding within the space of two months. The monthly flow of blood was replaced with deep sadness and hot flashes that left me soaking wet with limp, soggy clothes clinging to my body, and torrents of tears. I was angry at things I thought I had forgotten about long ago. Actually, I had dismissed them when they had disturbed me, and unresolved, they had laid wait in my body to explode emotionally along side the hormonal changes of menopause. While this is probably an extreme example for most of you, there is likely some familiarity to the emotional and physical pattern if you are one of millions of women who have never had the opportunity to use Nature's gift as a time to examine what is not working in your life and "clean it out" or correct it.

Does Menopause have to be so uncomfortable? I don't think so. I believe our cultural assumptions about Menopause, coupled with our "throw away" attitudes and societal beliefs that we are only desirable when young, dispose us to expectations that Menopause will bring nothing but loss. Additionally, in our culture women have been valued most for their ability to bring forth children. This belief system still lurks in the subconscious of many of us, and the end of fertility signals a decline in self- esteem. Psychological belief systems and attitudes influence the intensity of menopausal symptoms. And seeing Menopause as a negative event has been, until recently, the most prevalent attitude in our culture. Thankfully, that is beginning to change, with writings of authors such as Christiane Northrup, Marianne Williamson, and Dianne Hales.

There is a reason Menopause has been named "The Change". Perhaps we should emphasize *The* rather than

Change, pointing out the momentous significance of stepping into all that we are as women and living our truth. It is at this point that women frequently get rid of everything that is not working in their lives and move into teaching others what they have learned. It is a time of queenly wisdom, where we can graciously bestow the fruits of our learning on the younger members of our kingdom or our community. Marianne Williamson believes that all women are queens, either potentially as we remember the truth of who we are, or realized queens, confident in ourselves. I believe her definition of queen cannot be improved upon:

"A Queen is wise. She has earned her serenity...she has suffered and grown more beautiful because of it. She has proven she can hold her kingdom together. She has become its vision. She creates order where there was none. She cares deeply about something bigger than herself. She rules with authentic power" (33).

For nine years I was given the task of raising a child who sometimes called me "Queen Rebecca." In return, I dubbed her "Empress" and did my best to bring out her own divine nature. I welcomed the opportunity to guide her, and even more importantly, to grow with her as we moved into relationship. I was certainly a queen in potential back then, rather than a realized one, and I believe the child's vision held "what was possible," combined with an intense longing for a Queen Mother to guide and direct her at a young and tender age. However, her continued reference to me as Queen Rebecca kept me at task to recognize the divinity within myself, to live up to it, and to become a real queen. Ultimately, that task required that I leave the family to save myself. Yet I am deeply grateful for the child's vision of me, as well as the challenges she gave me. I learned a great deal as I struggled towards becoming a queen. She taught me how to let go my own beliefs, to suspend judgment, and look beyond what you "know," to see the validity in doing something differently; she taught me to see the beauty and grace in acceptance and to listen for things that are not spoken; her trust of me was a gift larger even than her love.

So was I a queen? Am I a queen? I would say that I was a queen in the making, and as someone now somewhat further along on the path, I would tell all awakening queens that the first kingdom we must learn to rule is our own inner territory. It is imperative that we learn to accept *what is* with dignity and grace, that we stand up for our rights and our needs with integrity, that we do not fold in the face of conflict, that we live from authenticity, and that we do not allow our desire for love to lead us into acquiescence or poor choices that do not honor who we are as queenly beings.

It seems very plain to me that Menopause can be a time when we have blossomed into all that we can be, if we have done our work. Menopause can be a crowning of the queen, as we step forward to rule from a place of wisdom. We can choose to step into our power as our lifeblood is rerouted to strengthen our very bones. We can wake from the sleepy forgetfulness that has compelled many of us to mourn our cycles rather than celebrate them. We can look back and be glad. Now we can rearrange the view imposed by society. We no longer have to accept the patriarchal beliefs that demoted our passions to a mere offering of fertile grounds for giving birth to sons.

Once we have rearranged our view, we can use the journey we have made to create a different path for our daughters. It is at this point that we have something to teach. It is only when we have acquired such knowing and acceptance of ourselves for who we are and put away childish competitions or untoward desires to be other than we are, that we deserve to wear the crown. It is only then that we can, by ruling our inner kingdoms, shine the light of peace and love into our outer kingdoms. We step into the role of wise queen who knows and can guide the wisdom of the blood, for we now carry it within us, and we can direct its power as we choose.

Our whole lives have lead up to the moment we cross into Menopause, like a bud opening to full flower. Menopause is that magical time when wisdom flows instead of blood, when many experiences of Nature's gift crown us with glory of all we have been, all we have learned, all we have done. *Now* we can teach. Now we can share from a place of wisdom. Now we can truly know the power of what it is to be a woman, if we have done our work on ourselves along the way.

If we have ignored our own work, our own whisperings of what needed to be attended, what needed to be left behind, what needed to be completed, then the winds of Menopause can bring torrents of change, rather than the gentle murmurs of new directions. Every cycle we have had has culminated in this moment, the moment that we either unleash the fury of unheeded impulses towards health in a deluge of emotional and physical uneasiness, or we fully understand the glory of being a woman and step forward to be crowned queen.

Menopause is an opportunity. Menopause is a time of emptying and refilling. It is *The* Change! So, don't sweat the hot flashes, if you have them. Smile at the river of fire that courses through you as you come into a new place of balance. Be willing to take your sweater on and off a few times as your inner thermostat regulates to this new climate. When you are angry or distraught, use the anger or sadness that wells up to fuel the necessary changes. If you have never listened to your body, *start now.* The emotions that are demanding attention need to be heard. If you have never experienced Nature's gift as a sacred time, a time apart to listen, cleanse what is not working, and create new harmonies in your life, you will need to go inward during Menopause to listen, really listen.

After you have listened to your body, spoken with your own shadow in the dark, sat with your own disappointments and heartaches, grieved your losses, and healed your heart, you will be ready to use the emotions you feel to speak against injustice. Be a champion for the Earth. Teach our daughters and granddaughters how to honor the extraordinary blessing of cycling with Nature, washing away what is not needed every month to purify the vessel, then in the quiet of Nature's gift, incubating what is to be, taking the seeds that are planted during this magical time after the flood to nurture them in the fertile ground we have created by allowing the process and participating with it. Teach all our children how to come back into balance.

Above all, honor the fact that you are a woman and that you have done the very best you knew how to do in any given moment, whatever that has been. We learn how to be better from experiences where we did not do all that was possible. We cannot change the past but we can change the present. By changing the present, we change the future to better match our dreams. Remember, Menopause is about change. So, *change*!

Best of all, remember that there is wonder in being a woman who has attained the wisdom of listening to what her body has to tell her. It is time to demonostrate our power as we move into the magical time after the flood. Menopause is the time to nurture new ideas, new projects, and yes, even new life, in the fertile ground we have prepared by allowing the process and participating with it. Menopause gives us the opportunity to step into being a queen, to teach our daughters to *Cleanse, Listen, Incubate, and Bloom.* They do not know the power they hold for changing the world. Let us, as queens, begin to teach them.

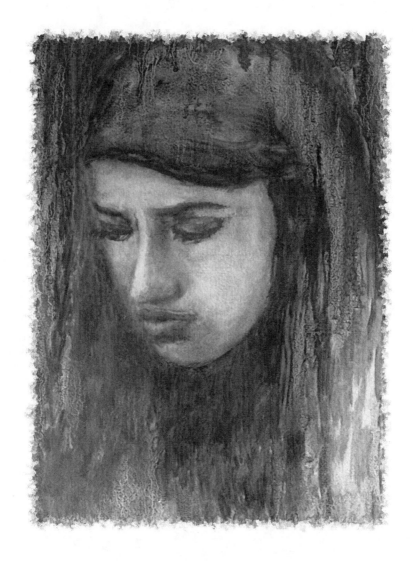

ANOTHER CHANCE
—Rebecca Smith Orleane

Another Cycle
　　Another Chance
Round and Round
　　　I move with the Dance

THIRTEEN:

THE RETURN OF DIVINE FEMININE: MARY ENERGY

Long before I studied the effects of the cycles in science class, long before I skipped along the ocean shore as the tide flowed in and out, long before I felt my own tides coursing through my body every month, I understood a divine feminine presence within Nature. Yet the myths of my culture overpowered my own inner knowing.

Joseph Campbell spent his life studying worldwide myths and how those myths affected people's interaction in daily life. He proposed that myths are designed to put our way of life in accord with Nature. Yet the myths alive within our current culture seem to *separate* us from Nature. Our existing myths have left us constantly seeking to correct an imbalance we know intrinsically is wrong. Our myths have given our children a legacy of confusion. Gender roles and gender interactions are desperately out of balance, leaving our girls trying to act like boys and our boys oblivious of the merit of unpredictability. How have we allowed our myths to define who we are? If we don't like the effects of our myths, we must change them and rewrite mythical instructions. Change of this magnitude requires relinquishing cherished beliefs and learning instead to trust our inner knowing. The divine feminine is reawakening, and She is calling us to listen to the truth of who we are.

A good beginning for returning to the divine feminine calls for us to re-educate our young about sexual exchange. Young women today are as confused as young men about sexuality, along with everything else. In the fight to be more like men, women have relinquished their native guidance about the appropriate sharing of sexual connection. Our culture promotes an appalling casualness about sex that leaves our children bereft of the joys of true and deep connection. I am not speaking about the Christian ethic of "saving oneself for marriage," which comes from a feudal system based on ownership. I am speaking of inner guidance that goes beyond hormonal drives in determining when and with whom to connect sexually, the guidance of the heart that leads to sharing the body only when deep love is present. The confusion about the way sexual exchange occurs in our culture shows a real loss of the feminine principle. Life always shows a biological imperative that drives men to spread their semen into as many women as possible to ensure the continuance of human life. The biological imperative of women has always been to encourage and direct containment of sexual activity in order to promote family and to insure a safe, nurturing environment for children to grow. The sacred responsibility of women is to govern sexual exchange through love.

Beyond biological imperatives and social competition for equality, the larger human understanding of depth and commitment in relationship has been all but lost in today's confusing social mores. Movement away from and attempts to control Nature have promoted existing imbalances and outright denial of beneficial and healthy natural tendencies, further harming our environment and our relationship with Earth. The imbalance is clearly reflected in rising promiscuity of both women and men. The idea of sex to "feel good" or for shallow fun is eroding the possibility of any depth of communication between genders and forcing many of our young people into an hardened roles of anticipated failure, a sort of "get what you can because nothing lasts" attitude that derails the very foundation of possibility. The women's lib movement and other feminist philosophies have twisted female-male interaction away from Nature in a misunderstood striving for "equality". It is unwise and naïve for women to hold the philosophy of "what is good for the goose is good for the gander" in their sexual understanding. Sexually transmitted diseases are on the rampage, unwanted children are pouring onto an already severely overburdened planet, abortions leave young girls scarred and confused or feeling victimized rather than powerful about their choices, and families are a dying concept.

Media and movies, magazines, even government, promote certain lifestyles, filling the heads of our young people with notions of instant romance and the "right to leave if it doesn't work," so that the notion of actually *working through* difficult situations to obtain better understanding and true connection is disregarded in favor of the internet-me-generation "I deserve this *now*" formulaic approach to life. We, as a culture, are creating a generation of narcissists who are concerned about others only for appearances sake, are disconnected from not only the cares of others but also from their own hearts, and certainly hold no reverence for the life of the planet that sustains and supports them. We need to change our views about life, and the beginning of change is to relinquish old belief systems and rewrite the myths that define our reality. The myths that govern us today were largely born out of or influenced by patriarchal ideas exemplified within the Christian church. As already discussed, these myths have placed women in a subordinate position. Internet and the transmission of instant information is supporting the confusion about sexual exchange as well, for it is the common belief among many young people that they deserve instant gratification, instant receiving of whatever they want, including orgasms and human connection. It can't and doesn't happen quite like that, but many of our young people in this poor confused generation are caught in an illusion that they are living the good life, having a good time, and are experiencing true freedom, while the deeper yearnings within them rot the possibility of becoming who they are or sharing with true heart. The return of the feminine requires that we begin to listen from the heart again and remember the value of women in our world.

An important first task for rewriting women's place in the world is to honor women as beings who are blessed with one of Nature's cycles every month. A second task is to live in a way that we set good examples for our daughters, teaching them the wonder and power of their own cycles and how to honor themselves as women. These two actions alone would create new myths and form a new set of instructions for our daughters and our sons. With women no longer setting the example of cycling as part of Nature, humans have abandoned natural human rhythms and adopted artificial rhythms of life. Because modern people are ignoring many natural biological rhythms (for example not honoring circadian rhythms while working at night, or not resting during menstruation), we are a long way from feeling or understanding the degree of harm we are causing our environment and ourselves. Women particularly suffer, struggling to survive in an environment that demands they continually adapt their natural rhythms to an artificial schedule. Additionally, the acceleration of rhythms in day to day living adversely affects people's nervous systems. These effects can be seen in the mounting numbers of physical and emotional maladies, many of which are more prevalent in women, who are more severely affected by ignoring Nature's pleas. Emilie Conrad says that we are allowing a mechanistic way of living to endanger our lives as bio-humans; in short, our love affair with machines at the cost of valuing our natural rhythms is about to cause our extinction.

Worldwide indigenous myths about menstruation tell us that having a monthly cycle is not a "curse", but rather a beautiful representation of how to live our lives within Nature's flow. The real "curse" in Western patriarchal society is the unrealistic valuing of constancy. Our youth are trained to be consistent in their performance, and the only change welcomed in the work force is increased productivity. Being a constant producer is valued. Having a monthly "down time" (with accompanying introspection) is not. Entering into quietude is discouraged as non-productive, and women who do so are often considered "moody" or anti-social. This negative view of inner retreat at the expense of outer productivity is what we model for our children, beginning at birth.

As women, we sometimes feel ineffective in managing our lives according to the linear patriarchal guidelines of our culture. We generally feel awkward varying our work or home routines according to where we are in our menstrual cycle. We want to make a difference, but we often feel our natural inclinations are discounted as frivolous, irrelevant to material progress, or just plain wrong. Natural contributions are often thwarted by the necessity of conforming to artificial rhythms of synchronized calendars and artificial electric lights, rather than following the rhythms and natural lighting of day and night. Unlike our ancestors who lived in harmony with the cycles of Nature rather than trying to control them, we live with artificial man-made timing, following prevailing myths that spurn the wisdom of the body. Our cultural myths perpetuate our treating menstruation as something to be "dealt with" or simply ignored. Menstruation is treated as an inconvenience. Because we frequently must adhere to the synthetic rhythm of our culture, the time we set aside for our most precious inspirations is designated to nights and weekends, when we may to be too tired to do anything but rest.

How can we move from a weakened position to a position of power within our culture? If our myths don't support belief in our gifts, how do we influence an environment that continually harms us? As already pointed out, women today are subject to becoming unbalanced through hormones in food, toxins in air and water, too hurried a pace, and society's demands to be what we are not. Is it any wonder that today's women often are more depressed or anxious, or more prone to addictions of all kinds, both overt and hidden? Is it any wonder that today more women are angry, more out of control, and more violent? The number of women in jail in the small county where I worked while writing this book increased in only a few years from five women inmates to sixty women inmates at any given time. I offered volunteer counseling sessions for some these distraught women, who were angry from not only having lost their sense of where they belong in the world, but were bereft of wisdom about who they were. They lost a sense of balance within themselves, and this imbalance reflected in the actions that land them in jail.

I see the evidence of repressed anger in my clients every day. Unaddressed, unresolved anger that surfaces pre-menstrually in women who have no understanding of the mechanism of Nature's gift as an opportunity to purge and change, is disconcerting to both the woman experiencing the anger and those around her. Both men and women are frightened of what has been called PMS rage, and rightly so. Anger that builds uncontrollably and has no direction is harmful. It can become explosive and even violent, either verbally or physically. That kind of anger destroys relationships and eventually destroys the self, leaving cinders of regret and waves of guilt for inappropriate behavior. The woman who is angry every month and doesn't understand why, or who doesn't know how to use her anger for positive change, hurts herself and everyone around her. The perceived split between her "normal, sweet, giving, going-along-with-everything" self to the "crying, raging, unhappy-with-everything" self takes its toll. There is no balance. What she seeks but does not understand is the natural flow between giving to others and turning inward to nurture herself. Doing versus Being. Being Active versus Intuiting and Understanding. If she is constantly in the mode of action, eventually she will get caught in Reaction and possibly Overreaction. There is no space for clearing, introspection, intuition, guidance, and creative solution.

A very good starting point for updating our myths and changing the paradigm about women's value is to address the cultural assumptions surrounding women's important natural cyclical process. We need to really examine how our current myths encourage us to act during this sacred time. Cultural biases are imbedded at an unconscious level, and they affect everyone. The television and magazine advertisements insisting that women can continue doing everything the same way, even during menses lead women to believe they *should* continue their daily routine. This media-reinforcing pressure leads us to deny our dual natures. The artificiality of expecting each day in a woman's monthly cycle to be the same is, as I have said, a further separation from Nature. Is this the best way to honor the gift of our biology?

We need to start thinking about these things and consider other possibilities. Walt Whitman was known to say, "Very well, then, I contradict myself; I am large, I contain multitudes." Why not adopt this attitude as a way of dealing with assaults on our dual nature? Reclaiming the gifts of having a dual nature and awareness of the positive benefits of having a monthly cycle are equivalent to taking back our voice and power. It is time to re-discover the value of tuning in to our introspective, intuitive, creative side. We simply *must* honor this powerful time that occurs once a month. If we fail to treat the gift of change with respect and honor, the gift becomes a nightmare (PMS, relationship problems, depression, other health problems) rather than a sacred dream (inspiration, creativity, harmony). Nature has given us a gift of time set aside to expel the old and make room for the new. We need to learn to *use* it properly. Slow down, empty, and expel what is not needed. Cleanse, ask for guidance, and *wait*. It is not the time to "do". The doing will be accomplished more efficiently and quicker when the time and space to receive guidance and conceive creative ideas has been honored.

I have throughout this book encouraged women to withdraw during Nature's gift. Some women may find that they enjoy the retreat so much that they continue separation and coming together in a rhythmic manner even after their own bleeding has stopped. For me, the duality of extremes in cyclic separation and return are no longer necessary in my life in the same way. I don't know if it is because I passed into menopause with a greater understanding of how to listen, or if it is finally being fully in relationship with the only person who is right for me, or both. But whatever the reason, our separations hold more unity than separateness, and I feel the balance offered through his maleness even when we are apart.

Our times of togetherness are closer, richer, deeper, on *all* levels, than I ever knew was possible when I was a younger woman. I am blissfully blessed in my relationship, and whatever we are experiencing together or separately is just right for that moment. We are spiraling together in life, through life, and I find myself no longer needing to withdraw to my cave to re-nurture myself. I am not advocating that women aspire to this type of connection while they are still having menstrual cycles, for as long as the magic of cycles is present, retreating to listen to their own inner guidance is necessary. What I am suggesting is that a real honoring of our cyclic duality may automatically move us towards a cosmic spiral of greater unity and greater connection within our relationships. Everything is possible when we work with Nature instead of trying to control Her. We need to teach our husbands and our sons, who have their own natural rhythms, as well as our daughters, to respect and understand the intuitive wisdom that comes from following these natural rhythms. Nothing but greater harmony will come from understanding that flexibility and adaptability create balance. Nature is not static. We are part of Nature. We have seasons as well---times to be dormant and times to bloom. In honoring this, we honor all of creation.

In a modern practice of honoring the menstrual cycle, we must learn the importance of withdrawing to clear a space from the filters that normally color our perception. We must give ourselves a quiet space in which to listen, and give our guidance an opportunity to speak. *All things manifested in this world originate with a dream, a vision, or a thought.* Out of these times of deep listening and power, the potential harmony of the world is born. It is in our power to "dream up" a million ways to make a difference. It is our sacred responsibility to listen and bring ways to heal to the world.

If we understand the necessity and value of deep listening, we can teach our children to be better listeners ourselves. The first step is to listen to our bodies. Our girl children need to know how to listen to the tides that course through them. Our male children also need to learn how to listen to their own bodies: to work or play when they are inspired, to rest when they are weary. By watching us, they may learn to listen better to themselves. Listening enhances communication. Better communication enhances relationships. Our relationships are all in trouble, from our relationships with ourselves to our relationship with Earth. Divorce is on the rise, and split families are the norm in Western culture. Worst of all, we are filled with our own shadows and unable to find peace within ourselves. We need creative vision of a new way of being in relationship- *all* relationships. We need to model for our children a better way to relate. Without proper times of retreat, creativity has no room to grow.

As we change our existing myths and create new ones, we can create a new reality. If you are puzzled about how to do this, simply look at what is not working in your life and imagine how it could be different. The imagination is a wonderful gift we can use as a tool to dream our way towards action. Once you can see what you want to change, you can start to make it happen. Stop believing in old ideas and accept the wisdom of your heart in imagining new possibilities. Incorporating new ways of doing things a little at a time can make a bigger difference in our lives than we realize. We just have to do one little thing at a time, listening to our hearts, and dream our way to where we want to be.

In our modern day experience of the world, many of us are too busy, too distracted, too hungry for something we need, or just plain trying too hard. It may seem overwhelming to begin to make changes, so I will offer a few practical suggestions for creating a new reality: The most valuable suggestion I can offer is to *slow down.* Create the opportunity to listen deeply. Find your own connection to Nature and honor it. Re-establish respect for your own inner rhythms. To explore possibilities, you may want to experiment with setting up your own private sacred space to cleanse and dream and connect with spiritual guidance. If you have a partner, be sure he understands and supports your exploration. It is not helpful in relationships to suddenly leave the marital bed without clearly explaining your intention. Additionally, if your partner feels rejected or abandoned, it will be more difficult for you to focus on your own exploration. A thoughtful and kind explanation can give both of you an opportunity to grow as you explore this path. Design your own sacred space to feel comfortable and inspiring to you. Make it inviting and soothing. Include candles, fresh flowers, special art or objects, favorite books, a journal, crayons or paints, whatever you want that inspires you. Put in tissues in case you decide you need a good cry. Decorate in colors that induce reflection. In that space, incubate your ideas and emerge from your sacred space with a creative plan to incorporate positive changes in your life. Put yourself first, for a change. How can you help all the people who depend on you if you don't take care of yourself? Rest.

Write your thoughts and feelings in a journal, as if you were writing to a special friend. Paint or dance your emotions. Carve out time to spend with someone special you rarely see but long to. Stop the same old arguments you always have. Change your beliefs. Give up trying to convince someone else of your viewpoint and honor the fact that you can be right for yourself alone. Start your own savings account to make your dreams come true. Plan (then take) a trip you have always wanted to take. Dream and acknowledge your dreams- the day and the night kind. Keep a dream journal by your bed and record the guidance that comes through in your sleep. Color in it. Keep a mood chart and see how often you are peaceful and content. If you find you don't spend much time feeling content, look at what is happening in your life when you are feeling sad or angry or just plain tired. Change it.

Chart your own rhythms: When do you feel sensitive and

quiet? When do you seek the company of others? When do you feel creative? When are you more intuitive? When do you solve problems easier, and when do problems overwhelm or tire you? When is your sex life the richest? When do you find it easiest to communicate clearly with your partner? With your children? With your friends? At work? Color your chart and make it a personal reflection of your own inner rhythms. Recognize the ebb and flow of going inwards and of wanting to connect. It is a natural gift to have the dual nature of doing both.

Learn to be grateful for the times you are more sensitive and cry more easily, for these are windows to see what is out of balance and needs to change. Learn to honor the right time for the right action, or inaction. Fully experiencing Nature's gift does not mean becoming weak or being restricted from doing something. Neither is PMS an excuse to be emotionally out of control. A sacred retreat during Nature's gift is about listening to your inner wisdom in order to know *when* is the most appropriate and most effective time to do what your visions and dreams show you, to make a special project *really* work, to help your family and community, to make a difference in the world. Rhythms of life bring Change. If we listen well, we can direct that change for a better world.

For now, I want to encourage a beginning step, a step for the health of women, families, and the planet Herself. I encourage women to slow down from their daily activities, or rest, during the time they are bleeding. Resting during menstruation not only gives the physical body a chance to cleanse and heal, it offers the benefit of allowing a woman's attention to gravitate to spiritual planes to gather wisdom. For those who do want to try separation during Nature's gift for spiritual, creative, or relationship benefits, be gentle with your first efforts in this direction. Remember that even if we do not use this sacred cleanse to prepare for new life, retiring to listen to spiritual guidance brings greater harmony as a result of ideas, solutions, brainstorms, and inspiration that arrive through dreams. The portal is wide open during this time, when we need to be in our own space, free of distracting influences.

Ask any woman what is important in her life, and very likely she will speak of the importance of relationships, intuition, creativity, dreams, and spirituality. Honoring the dual nature of being female enhances all of these areas. Additionally, following Nature's plan to retreat, cleanse, listen, dream, and then create enhances each of these areas. Yet, interestingly, these are areas that most often get ignored in the rush of contemporary Western living. We recognize that these areas are important, not only to us, but also to our families, our communities, and ultimately to the world, yet we find little time to enhance them.

In my opinion, withdrawing to a quiet space alone on a regular basis gives our guidance an opportunity to be heard. A room of our own, a quiet walk alone in Nature, or any special place where we can feel connected is appropriate. The place is important, and so is the timing. Out of these power times are born the harmony of the world. These suggestions are individual ways that we can make a difference in our lives by honoring our own needs as women. To reinstate an ancient practice of viewing menstruation as a spiritual retreat requires small steps to gain acceptance in modern culture and, if such a large-scale change were to come about, it would change every aspect of the way all of us live. It is in our power to "dream up" a million ways to make a difference. And it is our sacred responsibility as women to listen and bring ways to heal the world.

We have explored the beauty and meaning of cycles throughout this book, coming to understand that cycles represent life. We cycle through everything; we spiral as we grow and change and move. Yet the purpose of the polar opposites we cycle through is to show us that **we cannot be whole without accepting all of who we are, and we cannot find Unity until we learn to see that each part, no matter how different, has beauty and contributes to the whole.** This understanding reflects divine feminine consciousness.

Divine feminine energy has been represented by many images and names in different cultures. Mother Mary, Ishtar, Isis, Guadalupe, Shakti, Isanaklesh, and many others. I refer to it as "Mary energy," for that is how I experience it. The return of the feminine is reflected in an increase of Mary's energy being felt on Earth. Mary is the essence of the divine feminine. You can feel Her presence as love, for She represents opening the heart, and her presence is calling all of us to return to the realization that we are divine. The return of the Mary energy is a return to unity. The return to unity is the return of the feminine, for the feminine honors and respects the importance of every aspect of the whole.

I believe we all wish the same wish to live in joy, in love, in health, and in peace. Mary's return calls us to wake up. The Mary energy is strong, and her voice is calling us to remember and recognize who we are and to reclaim our power. We can no longer allow others to control us, for we are part of the divine. We can no longer indulge in feelings of being "less than" or in actions that continually put others first before we can love and care for ourselves. We must love ourselves *first* before we can love others, for the love begins within *us*. Mary calls us to give birth to our true selves and to join the cycles of life from a place of divinity, recognizing the power we hold within our love. The secret is in love. We must continually allow the love to flow within us, out of us, and back to us.

The Mary energy is increasing, imploring us to honor the divine feminine in order to heal the imbalances of modern life. Is it possible that through our understanding of correct timing, our intuition, our insight, our listening skills, our dreams, and our creativity, *we* could be the ones who will save the world? It's up to us.

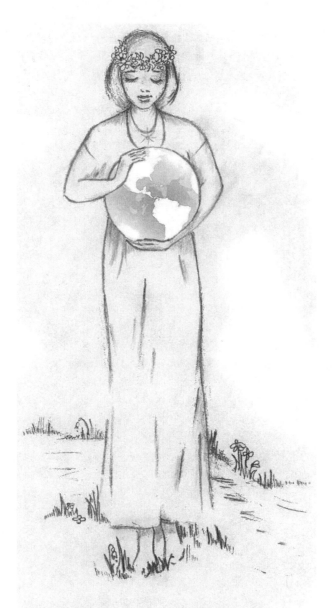

THE SACRED FEMININE
—Ron Russell

Mother Nature is another name
For the Sacred Feminine.
No one can ignore the Divine Feminine, as
She is the very source of life itself, and
We would not exist without her.

EPILOGUE

The time has never been more critical for returning to the wisdom of cycles. Feminine consciousness resides within all of us, yet has been suppressed by a linear culture. Linear thinking, focus on continual progress, increasing speed, and use of technology at the expense of integrating with our environment are causing further and further separation from Nature, the source of life.

In ancient times, women were responsible for leading us all towards balance so that harmony, peace, and health prevailed. As women have let go of their own values and picked up the values of men, our world has become more full of discord; war and illness far surpass health. The problem of imbalanced relationships (both personal and interplanetary) have grown large enough to require the full time attention of all of us, men and women. It is now up to all of us to get in touch with and listen to the call of the feminine within us, the call to return to natural cycles of balance, harmony, respect, and acceptance. The principles referred to in Chapter Two as principles of belonging are feminine principles, and all of us have a natural urging towards them. We want to belong; we want to connect. Yet our patriarchal culture has driven us to value things that have alienated us from Nature and our own natural rhythms, encouraging more and more separation rather than more and more connection. It is connection that we need, both as individuals and as part of a natural system of life on this planet.

I implore you to begin to notice how life is based on cycles. Notice the trees; notice the seasons; notice the cycles within your own moods and relationships. It is only when we begin to notice and understand the nature of cycles in life that we can see how out of balance we have become. It is egotistic to believe that we will always be a part of Earth. It is possible that if we separate ourselves enough from cycles of life, we can eliminate our own species. Ignoring, dismissing, or trying to control natural cycles, whether the cycles we ignore or try to control are sleep cycles, women's cycles, or cycles of weather, leads us further into delusions of control, and attitudes based on a need to control are most certainly related to separation, not connection. Life will not be controlled, for Nature has an intelligence of her own. Everything is connected, no matter how much we are deluded by our own narcissistic thinking.

If we continue to separate ourselves, we are destroying our own lives and the lives of our children.

A plea for the return of the feminine is a plea to save our own lives and the life of our planet. It is a plea to return to the wisdom of connection, grasping the understanding that everything cycles and that all cycles are connected and have importance for the whole. It is past time for breaking free from patriarchal dogma that has kept us imprisoned in dysfunctional beliefs about who we are and how we relate in the world. It is time that we turn around, look in the opposite direction, and honor and support the return of the feminine in order to save ourselves and save our world. Thank you for listening and doing your part.

CHAPTER NOTES

Chapter 3

1- Baker, R. (1980). The Mystery of Migration.

2- The Bible: Ecclesiastes 3:1-7

3- Thoreau, H. (2009). Civil Disobedience.

4- Eliade, M. (1954). The Myth of Eternal Return.

Chapter 4

5- Buckley, T. and Gottlieb, A. (1988). Blood Magic: The Anthropology of Menstruation.

6- Allen, P. (1986). The Sacred Hoop: Recovering the Feminine in American Indian Traditions.

7- Buckley, T. and Gottlieb, A. (1988). Blood Magic: The Anthropology of Menstruation.

8- Parker, K. (1993). Wise Women of the Dreamtime.

Chapter 5

9- Perdue, T. (1998). Cherokee Women: Gender and Cultural Change.

Chapter 6

10-Ford, G. (1996). Listening to Your Hormones.

11-Vliet, E. (1995). Screaming to be Heard.

12- Sichel, D. and Driscoll, J. (1999). Women's moods.

Chapter 7

13-Ogden, G. (2006). The Heart and Soul of Sex.

14-Kornfield, J. (1993). A Path With Heart.

Chapter 8

15- Ogden, G. (2006). The Heart and Soul of Sex.

16-Shuttle, P. and Redgrove, P. (1988). The Wise Wound: The Myths, Realities, and Meanings of Menstruation.

17-St. Pierre, M. and Long Soldier, T. (1995). Walking in the Sacred Manner: Healers, Dreamers, and Pipe Carriers- Medicine Women of the Plains Indians.

Chapter 9

18- Krippner, S. (2009). Extraordinary Dreams and How to Work With Them.

19- Achterberg, J. (1991). Woman as Healer.

Chapter 10

20- Conrad, E. (2007). Personal Conversation.

21- Runco, M. and Richards. R. (2009). Eminent Creativity, Everyday Creativity, and Health.

22- Ibid.

23- Ibid.

24- Ibid.

Chapter 11

25. Marks, W. (2001). The Holy Order of Water.

26. Gardner, R. (2004). Experimenting with Water.

27. Schwenk, T. (1989). Sensitive Chaos.

28. Paper, J. (1997). Through the Earth Darkly: Female Spirituality in Comparative Perspective.

29. Conrad, E. (2007). Life on Land.

30. Marks, M. (2001). The Holy Order of Water.

Chapter 12

31. Northrup, C. (2010). Women's Bodies; Women's Wisdom.

32. Ibid.

33. Williamson, M. (1993). A Woman's Worth.

Appendix B

34. Buckley, T. and Gottlieb, A. (1988). Blood Magic: The Anthropology of Menstruation.

35. Knight, C. (1991). Blood Magic: Menstruation and the Origins of Culture.

Appendix C

36. Bettelheim, B. (1955). Symbolic Wounds: Puberty Rites and the Envious Male.

37. Paper, J. (1997). Through the Earth Darkly: Female Spirituality in Comparative Perspective.

THE FIRST RULE
—Anonymous

Rule #1: You are unlike all others.

There is no Rule #2.

APPENDIX A:

THE RESEARCH

While pursuing my Ph.D. in Psychology at Saybrook University, I was searching for a topic for my dissertation. I had a very powerful dream, while exploring in my own life the territory of separation during Nature's gift. From that dream I decided to expand my exploration of separation during Nature's gift to possible experiences of other women during Nature's gift. The question I wanted answered was, "Does separate sleeping during a woman's menses affect her relationships, her dreaming, her creativity, or her intuition and spirituality?"

I designed and set in place a seven month study with Western women who had never been exposed to the idea of separate sleeping during menstruation. Requirements for participation included that each woman be in a monogamous heterosexual relationship of at least two years duration, that she be in good health with no known physical or mental concerns, that she have a space that could be turned into a "sacred space" for sleeping during menses, and that her partner be supportive of her participation in the research.

Finding volunteers was more difficult than I would have supposed. I posted announcements at health conferences and universities across the country. When I screened applicants, I found some who were interested but had not been with the same partner for the minimum time, some who had other complicating health issues, some who didn't want to sleep separately from their partners, some whose partners did not support their participation, and some who met all other criteria, but had no space. There were more women with reasons *not* to participate than volunteers who met all the criteria. That in itself was a profound statement to me about women's misunderstandings around the importance of all aspects of menstruation.

Finally, I had the required number of volunteers in place; it was a small but noteworthy number for a preliminary study that turned out to be ground-breaking work. In two years of researching existing literature, I did not find any other studies of this type. The women who participated in the research came from varied backgrounds, including geographical locations, age, education, and spiritual practices. While I preferred to include in the study only women without PMS, it was impossible to do so because, without exception, every woman interviewed answered affirmatively the question ""Do you have PMS?" Women who listed only the mildest premenstrual changes, such as bloating, breast swelling, headaches, abnormal appetite or food cravings, fluid retention, acne, headache, and heightened emotions attributed these changes to Premenstrual Syndrome, rather than understanding that increased sensitivities and changes are a normal part of the female cycle. At final selection, only women who experienced normal monthly changes, as those listed above, were chosen.

The protocol for the study required that each woman arrange a sacred space in her house to which she could retire at any time of her choosing and where she would sleep during menses for five months. In the first and seventh months of the study, each woman slept with her partner as usual in order to compare the effects of the five months they slept separately during Nature's gift.

Each participant was given a journal and instructed to write or draw in it daily. All events significant to each woman were to be recorded, including dreams, relationship issues, spiritual experiences, and creative ventures. If nothing significant happened in their lives, they recorded that. The women were also given questionnaires and instructed to fill them out on the first day of bleeding in the first, fourth, and seventh month. Responses were counted and tracked for change over time. Finally, each woman was interviewed in the first, fourth, and seventh month, and their partners were interviewed at the end of the study.

My research focused on the cyclical process of women's lives, and the effects of treating menstruation as a sacred time for withdrawing for contemplation and experimentation with separate sleeping during this most potent time. I hoped I would discover beneficial effects on creativity, dreaming, intuition, and relationship harmony that would help women. Indeed I did!

The possibilities were explored with women volunteers who were willing to commit to the practices and reflection required during the seven month duration of this study. Empowering effects were hypothesized for each of the four areas traditionally important in women's lives. I examined, in a contemporary Western context, the effects of treating menses as a sacred time, as has occurred throughout history in various indigenous traditions. A key aspect of sacredness in many traditions is separate sleeping during menses, a practice believed to bring deeper insights from dreams, more creativity in day to day affairs, more harmony in home and community, and deeper connection to spiritual and intuitive guidance.

Below are the questions I posed in my research, and a brief summary of the results for each question:

1. <u>Will Women Who Sleep Separately During Menses Experience Increased Creativity?</u>

The research showed that the women in this study

experienced a general increase in creativity overall from the first month to the seventh month, and many of the women began to have a greater urge to create or developed more creativity towards the end of each period of menstrual retreat.

2. <u>Will Women Who Sleep Separately During Menses Experience Greater Dream Recall?</u>

The research showed *all of the women* (100%) reported greater dream recall over the course of the seven months, increasing each month from the first month until the end of separate sleeping. Women who were unaware that they even dreamed were astounded to discover that they not only dreamed, but that they began to remember their dreams during the course of the research.

3. <u>Will Women Who Sleep Separately During Menses Experience More Meaningful Dreams?</u>

The research demonstrated *all of the women* (100%) reported an increase in meaningful dreams. Most of the women divulged that their most meaningful or powerful dreams occurred during menses or just immediately before menses *when they were sleeping separately during Nature's gift,* although there was some variation. Women who were unaware that they even dreamed at all began to have dreams that carried meaning into their everyday lives. They were using these dreams, which they considered spiritual dreams, for guidance by the end of the research. Additionally, 95% of the women reported a decrease in dreams or an increase in disturbing dreams when they returned to their shared beds in the seventh month; one woman was stung by a wasp, which she interpreted as an indication that she was sleeping in the wrong place at the wrong time.

4. <u>Will Women Who Sleep Separately During Menses Have More Spiritual Experiences?</u>

All of the women reported a keen awareness of their spirituality during the research. Half the women reported being more aware of spirituality, while the other half noted a marked increase in daily spirituality in their lives. All of the women reported that spirituality was a general undercurrent that was present in every part of daily living by the end of the research. A third of the women were drawn more to spiritual issues during menses. Every women reported being more content with life, more aware of and connected to her inner guidance, and having belief changes by the end of the research period.

5. <u>Will Women Who Sleep Separately During Menses Experience Increased Intuitive Experiences?</u>

All the women in the study reported that their intuition increased by the end of the research. Half of the women linked their intuition to incubating creative ideas, which they acted on later. Half of the women connected their increased intuition to an increase in spirituality. A third of the women felt their intuition was stronger during menses, and all of the women reported that their intuition was more active during the entire month by the end of the study.

6. <u>Will Women Who Sleep Separately During Menses Experience Increased Relationship Harmony?</u>

This question received a resounding Yes! from both participants and their partners. Women who were struggling with long term unresolved issues reported resolving the problems; women who had experienced unexpressed anger with their partners for years learned to express it and express themselves; partners reported clearer communication; sex lives improved; both participants and their partners reported decreased conflict and quicker conflict resolution; both told stories of increased "personal moments," more satisfying intimacy, and deepening of their relationships. All women said they were glad that they had participated in the research, and many planned to continue the practice of menstrual separation after the research was finalized.

The reason for having three ways to gather data was to be sure nothing was left out or misunderstood. For example, one woman who checked "fine" for every question about relationship on her questionnaire and had only good things to say about her spouse poured out her heart in her journal about being lonely and misunderstood in her marriage. Another woman who found it difficult to write her feelings in her journal, filled the questionnaire with side comments and remarks about her life.

Quantitative and qualitative data of this research yielded statistically significant results at a level less than .03 percent in all four areas of questioning. What that means is that, according to strict scientific standards, the positive results I obtained could not be attributed to *chance*.

When I began my research, I did not expect that long-term effects could be seen until more time had passed because it was the first study of its type. However, the effects turned out to be more far reaching than expected. My hope by presenting my research in a more "user friendly" version in the form of this book, is to reinstate time honored understanding of the many gifts of being a woman. If we recreate the myths that have constricted us, if we are true to our natures and begin to live out of our truth, we have the potential to change the world.

For those readers who would like more information or verification of constructs presented in this book, you may order my 2001 original dissertation: <u>Empowerment of Women Through Sacred Menstrual Customs: Effects of Separate Sleeping During Menses on Creativity, Dreaming, Relationships, and Spirituality</u>.

Order from:

ProQuest

300 N. Zeeb Road

Ann Arbor, MI48106-1346

Be sure to include title, year of publication (2001) and sponsoring university, (Saybrook University) in your request. You will find detailed support of many of the contentions presented in this work.

CHANGE
—Rebecca Smith Orleane

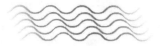

Five letters in B-L-O-O-D,
Five letters in P-O-W-E-R,
Five letters in H-O-N-O-R.
Five is the number of CHANGE.

How will I greet you, CHANGE,
As you come knocking at my door?
Though HONORING the POWER
And the rhythm of my BLOOD.

APPENDIX B:

TABOS SURROUNDING MENSTRUATION

Because of the intense beliefs surrounding blood, particularly menstrual blood, it easily follows that some sort of rules were needed to contain or control the power contained in menstrual blood. One word recurs again and again across cultures: *taboo*. The word taboo, or tabu, is made up from the root ta, meaning 'to mark', and pu', which is an adverb of intensity. Taken together, *tapua* (a Polynesian word) means "sacred" and "menstruation". In English, the word is translated as *taboo*.

The most commonly found taboos across cultures have to do with menstruation. Throughout history, taboos surrounding menstruation developed into laws that were enforced, sometimes, to the point of death. Again, this reveals belief that menstruation holds deep power that must be contained or controlled, thus leading to the belief that women had to be controlled or contained. When men understood that women had the power to create life, and that this power was connected to menstruation, they made a connection to death as well and began to fear women's power. It was at this point that men decided to disempower women, to constrain and control them, and to find a way to take the power they held. Taboos around menstruation were created by women who understood the power contained in the mysteries of menstruation and by men who wished to control that power. While the origination of taboos is marked with controversy, I contend that the Christian Church was a very big player in this scheme, creating a myth that spelled out the danger of listening to women's wisdom and punishing them for bringing forth life. Bearing in mind the fact that most early research on taboos was done by men, it is not surprising to find a universal myth of the toothed vagina as a source of an incredible number of taboos on menstrual blood. The toothed vagina is symbolic of a recognized power held in the blood, capable of harming a man.

Taboos originating prior to the Christian Church can be traced to sacred observations leading to practices designed by women for women, practices women imposed on themselves and on men for the protection of all. Some anthropologists even went so far as to recognize that menstrual taboos indicated a superior status for women. For example, in

Portugal menstruating women set taboos in place because it allowed them to control certain social interactions and gave them a rationale for protecting the economic privacy of their homes, for which they held primary responsibility.

It is interesting to note that taboos surrounding menstruation originally restricted the behaviors of others more than the behaviors of the menstruating woman herself until the advent of Christianity. Each woman chose to seclude herself and avoid others. Interfering with her choice to remove herself from daily activities and interaction with others was forbidden. Only with the arrival of the Judeo-Christian ethics were women viewed as unclean temptresses to be strictly avoided. Through Judeo-Christian teachings, beliefs about menstruation as a powerful vehicle for change went underground and menstruation became something to be hidden, something shameful. If a woman were menstruating, she was seen as unapproachable, no longer because of her stance of power, but because of a taint placed upon her by the religion of her culture. No wonder it took women so long to publicly acknowledge the importance of one of their most primary bodily functions. Prior to Christianity taboos were devised to contain women's energies and keep them from spreading beyond a limited place in the order of things. Early menstrual taboos included separate sleeping during menses, food restrictions (including the fire which cooks food), non-touching, and avoidance of water, sunlight, and the earth. After Christianity the danger that came with women's monthly power was treated as something to contain rather than respect.

Separation taboos came into place for reasons already explained of protecting others from the potentially dangerous energy that surrounds the discharge of women's life-bearing blood. The reason for separation, unfortunately, was twisted until women became segregated with the stigma of being tainted or soiled, less holy than the men who condemned them. Contrary to recent history of separation taboos, early isolation of menstruous women, often in special shelters, was widespread in indigenous cultures. Yurok women did not sleep with their husbands during menstruation, nor engage in any regular daily activities. Menstruating women in Algonquian-speaking people of Labrador separated themselves in ceremony, sitting in an area sacred to women, opposite their husbands, an indication of separate, but equal gender positions. In many indigenous practices, ritual separation during Nature's gift is begun when a girl has her first menses, so she begins her marriage with the idea that menstruation is her sacred time and withdraws accordingly. Additionally, many indigenous societies have built-in social support that allows someone else in the family or community to take over a woman's duties during Nature's gift so that she can retire. Finally, many indigenous tribes have a cultural understanding of the underlying implications of a woman's power and how withdrawing during menses is appropriate for her own inner work, inspiration, and guidance for her community. In most tribes it was believed that until a woman (particularly young girls) learned how to control her energy it could be very dangerous. So their grandmothers took them to sacred women's lodges and taught them the ways of Nature's gift. Cherokee people acknowledged that a husband was affected by the power his wife was experiencing during Nature's gift because of the nature of their relationship. Therefore menstrual restrictions extended from her to him. Under no circumstances would a menstruating woman *or* her husband participate in a ceremony.

Menstrual lodges and sanctuaries were among the first features relinquished by native people upon Christian-European contact. While one might speculate that forced relocation of indigenous peoples by Europeans made it more difficult to maintain separate sleeping spaces for menstruating women, the more likely reason for the elimination of sanctified treatment of menstruating women (or *all* women) was that the treatment of menses in Christian-European patriarchal cultures was clearly different and more demeaning. The Wisdom Councils of many Native American tribes were actually made of women, who convened to discuss important issues, and from their discussions determined the actions the male chiefs would take for the benefit of the entire tribe. To conquer a powerful people, as all indigenous people were, the

Christian-Europeans began by disempowering the women. It could be said that the largest loss leading to the downfall of Native Americans in the United States was the loss of acknowledgment of their women's power. When that was displaced, it was easy to unbalance the culture and conquer the men. Men are nothing without the balance of women (and the same can be said for women; we need each other to be balanced).

Menstrual taboos around food and fire began pre-lingually. An ancient tribal tale tells of a collective sex strike orchestrated by the women of the tribe, who synchronized their monthly cycles and used their menstrual bleeding as a signal of "no!" when there was no food for the tribe. The absence of food and the response of no sex encouraged men to go off and hunt. Cooking and approaching fire for cooking as menstrual taboos makes sense, if one remembers that women who are discharging menstrual blood have great power. If a woman is discharging powerful emotions, it could energetically harm another who takes in the food prepared with such energy. Additionally, menstruation itself represents water and cold. Fire is hot. Water puts out fire, so why would an intelligent menstruating woman want to challenge the fire that cooks her family's food with the presence of her own very potent moisture? While most food and fire restrictions were in place because the power of the woman could overpower the life-giving benefits of the plant or animal, some food and fire restrictions were for the protection of the menstruant. According to the Anishnabe, berries were linked to the blood of the earth, so they were considered too powerful for a young girl to eat at a time when her own female powers were developing. Even today, among many indigenous tribes, cooking or approaching a cooking fire is a taboo that menstruating women observe. The Beng of Ivory Coast, do not cook or touch logs or coals of a fire while menstruating. Menstruating women of the Australian Arunta tribe do not gather the irriakura bulbs, a staple of their diet, lest the bulbs fail. Cherokee women do not farm, cook, or care for children during menstruation. In the Malekula and the Cherokee, the taboo extends from the menstruous woman to her husband; neither may enter a garden where young plants are growing. Other tribes worldwide have restrictions regarding the touching of certain, or all, foods during menstruation. It is thought that if one ingests food touched by a menstruating woman, the power internalized can cause severe harm. The power can also overcome and put out the fire that cooks the tribe's food, so menstruating women stay away.

With the arrival of Christianity in ancient Europe (and later in America) time honored food and fire taboos were twisted to demean menstruating women. In Rome menstruating women were avoided because of fables that they could turn wine sour, make crops barren, gardens dry, fruits fall off trees, hives of bees die, mirrors dim, and iron rust. Even today in Italy,

Spain, Germany, and Holland, peasants believe that flowers and fruit trees will wither from contact with a menstruating woman. The only difference in ancient and modern food taboos is the *attitude*, which has been colored from one of respect to one of rejection.

Other common ancient menstrual taboos concerned touch. Touch was considered a distracter from a woman's inner awareness. Sensual awareness was replaced by spiritual focus during menstruation. In many indigenous cultures, no one was allowed to touch a menstruating woman, nor would she touch herself or anyone else. Even scratching one's own skin or hair was prohibited during menstruation. A young Yurok woman explained this taboo against touch:

"A woman must use a scratching implement, instead of scratching absent-mindedly with her fingers, as an aid in focusing her full attention on her body by making even the most natural and spontaneous of actions fully conscious and intentional. You should feel all of your body exactly as it is and pay attention" (34). The taboo of non-touch during menses was used for gaining spiritual power. The discipline required to keep this taboo helped to create a person with strong mental concentration and great control of her own body. The issue of power kept the taboo of non-touch in place in most cultures. The Gimi of the Eastern highlands in Papua New Guinea believed menstruating women have such power that their touch would cause wooden bowls to crack, and stone axes to misbehave in the hands of their male owners, inflicting upon them otherwise inexplicable wounds (35). It was not only taboo to touch the living; sometimes this taboo extended to the dead. Among the Beng of Ivory Coast menstruating women are restricted from touching a corpse. Since the menstruating woman symbolizes fertility, she should not have close contact with a corpse, which is a symbol of death. Clearly this prohibition was in place to protect the woman.

Like touch, food, and fire restrictions, there were taboos around water and Earth for the protection of the menstruating woman. The Beng of the Ivory Coast would not set foot in the forest, protecting the menstruants from forces that were opposite of their own power. The Carrier Indians carried young menstruants bodily from point to point to keep their power separate from the earth. The Tiwi of North Australia believed a young girl's first bleeding caused her to be particularly vulnerable, and she honored many taboos for her own protection.

The separation from water and Earth probably came from a mythic belief that if menstrual blood mingled with Earth-blood (water), all of creation might unravel. Following this belief, menstruating women lifted the veil between one reality and another with the awareness inherent in the blood of life they carried and released through their bodies. With the understanding of how and why taboos were set in place, I trust each woman reading this work can find her own set of taboos to support and honor her own inner wisdom.

ODE TO WATER
—Dianne Windsong Martin ©2010

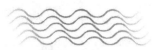

Oh the Water she is rushing
Cause the Mother is free,
Laughing and splashing on her way to the sea
Bubbling in the springs and over waterfalls
It's the blood of the Mother
As she nourishes all

Standing in the water
Water washing me clean
Healing sparkling water
Rushing over me

Give thanks to the water
Sing to the water
Pray for the water
Take care of the water

Mother Water Loves us
Mother Water Loves us
We are Water, we are Water, we are Water
Love the Water, Love the Water, Love the Water

APPENDIX C:

MENSTRUATION RITUALS AROUND THE WORLD

There are many stories about blood that created rituals throughout the world. The word ritual comes from R'tu, meaning any act of magic toward a purpose, and Rita, meaning proper course. R'tu has a secondary meaning of menstrual, suggesting that rituals perhaps first began in direct relation to menstruation. Whether or not the first rituals surrounded menstruation, rituals surrounding or involving blood have been a part of human history since pre-agricultural times. In hunting and gathering societies, both genders regularly came into contact with blood. For a man, it was the blood lost in the taking of life, either in hunting or in battle. For a woman, it was her own menstrual blood or the blood of childbirth. Both men and women considered anything to do with blood as dangerous.

The historical importance of blood shows itself repeatedly in art or in rituals. Ancient rock art showed the Maluti San collapsing in trance covered in blood pouring from the nostrils. The men in the dance are thought to have been expressing life-renewing ritual power. The earliest historically documented action occurring in a public forum was bloodletting. Classic Mayan art is full of bloodletting imagery. Ancient Mayan belief held that cutting the penis of the king induced trance and brought the gods into being. Connection between the ritual and the king's contact with the supernatural was clear. The cosmically potent ritual of kings was upheld as a form of menstruation: the king was the mother of the gods because he gave them birth and nourished them through his gift of blood.

Today we know through science that chemicals produced by the brain in response to massive blood loss (a form of endorphins) can induce hallucinogenic experiences. The Maya may not have understood how it worked, but they knew that drawing large amounts of blood would, without the help of other drugs, produce the visions they sought in their rituals. Through these bloodletting rituals and visions, the Maya brought the supernatural realm into the world of human beings.

Sub incision, slitting the penis along its length so that blood can drip over the man's lower body, is still practiced today in New Guinea, Australia, the Philippines, and

Africa. These cultures hold the belief that the blood flowing from the wound is no longer the man's blood but becomes sacred women's blood through ritual. Today Wogeo men of New Guinea believe women are automatically cleansed by menstruation. Since men do not have this automatic process, they periodically incise the penis and allow some blood to flow to cleanse themselves and to guard against potential illness. The Murngin and Dwoma of New Guinea also use this practice for cleansing. In each culture, this process is called "men's menstruation."

Historically, there were many parallel menstrual-like rites of seclusion and privation for Native American hunters prior to a hunting excursion, including special instruction by women elders, imitation of menstrual taboos, and induced visionary states. The men in tribal cultures modeled their own rituals as much as possible around the women's rituals. A man coming back from war, where he has seen blood, was not considered dangerous. However, he was often given a ceremony for cleansing and peace of mind. Today North American indigenous men participate in river plunges or sweat lodges for cleansing, acknowledging that ritual bleeding is for women only. Men see their own blood as less perilous than women's blood, which is still considered powerful and dangerous.

While men's rituals have historically attracted interest, in many cultures, men have not even been privy to women's rituals, and when they were, there was generally great respect for them. Only Western patriarchal society has frequently misunderstood women's rituals as something forced upon women. The misunderstanding comes, perhaps, from the inner truth outwardly denied by Christian European men: they *knew* the power inherent in women's bleeding and they intentionally set about to control that power by belittling it.

Other cultures throughout the world have varying approaches to rituals around blood. Some have no rituals for women; others offer rituals for the female with her entire family. In Japan, when a young woman begins her period, family and friends are invited for a celebration. While no reason for the celebration is given, candied fruit presented on a tray "candidly" tells the guests the reason for the celebration.

Cultures vary in deciding whether rituals are appropriate at the first menses only or are to be continued every time a woman is menstruating. In most indigenous cultures the world over, the first period is of such importance it is accompanied by rites that announce that the girl child has earned a woman's place in society. The seclusion of the menstruating girl from the tribe offers an opportunity for various women elders to explain to her the meaning and importance of ritual and what her responsibilities will be as a woman.

Menstrual blood is considered a gift by the Pygmies in central Africa. The entire community gratefully and joyously receives the gift with festivity. The girl who has reached menarche goes into seclusion, taking all her young friends with her. There, an older woman relative teaches them the arts and crafts of motherhood. A celebration lasting a month or two follows, and friends come from near and far to pay their respects.

In West Central Africa, Akan custom requires that a female who menstruates for the first time come out of her house at dawn crying. She then informs her mother, who gives her a white stool of honor on which to sit at the entrance of the house. The mother announces the news to the community, and older women assemble to sing special songs. The girl plants a peregun tree in the yard of her parents home. The mother pours wine to the spirits to ask for blessings for the girl; her hair is ritually shaved and preserved, symbolizing the death of her old state of life and rebirth into a new life. She is taken to the riverside, where a young girl and a young boy stand on her left and right, respectively. All three are immersed in the river three times, symbolizing the beginning, middle, and end of life and the appreciation for future birth of either a boy or a girl. White clay is smeared on her forehead, and she is taken home with her head covered. She is offered mashed yam three times, and she lets the food fall to the floor three times. Finally, a whole egg is touched to her mouth, which she rejects twice and swallows whole on the third time, signifying fertility and life.

In the Arunta and Ilpirra tribes of Africa, a mother

takes her daughter at first menstruation to a spot close to the women's camp, to which no man ever goes. The mother makes a fire and a camp and instructs the girl to dig a hole about a foot or eighteen inches deep. The girl then sits over this hole attended by her own and some other tribal mothers. "During the first two days she is supposed to sit over the hole without stirring away; after that she may be taken out by one or other of the old women hunting for food. When the flow ceases she is told to fill the hole. She now becomes what is called Wunpai, returns to the women's camp, and shortly afterward undergoes the rite of opening the vulva and is handed over to the man to whom she has been allotted" (36). Ritual similarities exist between present day African Arunta and ancient Anishnabe. In the past young Anishnabic women at menarche went to a specific vaginal shaped cave, understood to be the vagina of the Earth. There the girls sat listening to the nearby the creek, making the connection between the flow of their own bodies' blood and the flowing of the blood of Earth. I think this is a connection worthy of remembering for all of us, women *and* men. If we had more respect for the flow of women's blood and the understandings connected to it, we would, perhaps, also have more respect for the Earth. Neither the Earth's cycles, nor women's, need to be controlled. Each contains a natural power that supports the correct timing of life and death. Possibly it is recognition that women hold a deep understanding that everything has a correct timing, and death is part of the order, that causes so much fear and desire to control feminine cycles. If we understand that death comes when the time is right, we stand in the way of the men who defy death and seek to control what and who live and die. Looking at the world through wholly male eyes, we see an unending string of acts of death portrayed as supporting the progress of life: trees are cut and animals are slaughtered in their prime; wars are waged and lives are taken to preserve someone else's view of how life *should* be lived. More feminine views and understandings promote *all* life and a weaving and balancing of everything and everyone because everything is connected and the natural cycles of life and death are well understood.

In Aboriginal tribal life an older female, such as an aunt or grandmother, ritually guides young women through the initiatory experiences of menstruation and childbirth. For several months the young woman is covered with mud, smoked with special leaves, and able to eat only the food brought to her by her older female initiator. No sweets such as honey are allowed for four moons. After some time, the women of the tribe make her a camp closer to the big one. At that time she is painted with red ochre and white gypsum and adorned with sprays of sweet-smelling white flowers on her arms and head. White swans down is scattered over her head, and a sprig of a sacred tree is placed through the hole in the septum of her nose. The old woman gives her a bouquet of smoking leaves to carry as she walks toward the main camp. As she walks, the other women sing her songs in a strange language. The young woman then encounters her betrothed husband sitting on a log with his back to her. As the singing builds in a momentum and pitch, the young girl hurls her bouquet to the ground, grabs her betrothed husband on his shoulders, and shakes him. She then runs away. In a few weeks time, she is shifted again to a camp closer to the main camp. A fire is made for her, on the other side of which is camped her betrothed husband. This gradual bringing together of the couple increases the dramatic intensity and mystery surrounding their inevitable union.

The young couple camps like this for one moon, at the conclusion of which the old woman informs the young girl that it is time to camp on the same side as her husband as his wife. He is required to treat her well, or her relatives will take her from him. If we had such rituals in Western culture, courtships that honor natural timing and require respect from both parties with the support of family and community, would we see such shallow romances and so many divorces?

Anishnabic girls are immediately taken into the bush when their first menses begins. The girl makes a small shelter where she will stay until her bleeding stops. Her mother returns with necessities for her temporary residence. Each day a female elder spends the day with her, imparting the knowledge and sharing the wisdom she will need as an adult. She fasts for seven days. Girls usually have vision-dreams during this fast that empower them for the rest of their lives. The period of isolation is called makwa or "turning into a bear" (37). The Bear is a powerful healing spirit, closely connected with Earth. At the end of the fast, the girl, now woman, washes herself and her clothes and walks on a bed of cedar boughs for purification, then goes home for a ritual feast

Among the Dine, a kinaalda, meaning 'Blessing Way Ceremony', is performed for a young girl in honor of her first menses. Young girls in their first (or second) menstruations are considered to have a unique power that can bring positive effects to her family and tribe. To maximize these effects, families try to be prepared for the moment that the girl will inform her mother that her first menstrual period has begun. The bleeding is considered a sacred ceremony bringing blessings, and a blanket is hung over the Hogan, signifying that a ceremony is in progress. Blessing Way songs are sung among the Dine for the girl's first menses to counteract any danger to her or others that may be present. Legends of the first kinaalda tell the story of the girl running in joy on her own for four days, making up a new song each day. The songs gave her energy and prepared her for her existence. She ran with the songs in all four directions.

Following the legend of the first kinaalda, a new menstruant runs for four days, in the early morning, into good fortune. After running as far as she can, she stretches out her arms, takes four deep breaths, drawing in the dawn air with her arms each time. Then she bends down, touches Mother Earth, and blesses herself by applying moist soil to her body from her feet upward. Some of the reproductive power possessed by her during her first and second menses is transferred back to Mother Earth through this process. The final step in the ceremony after she runs and sings for four days is to be painted in white paint, recognition that she is symbolically the holy Dine Changing Woman. After her four-day ceremony, the young girl washes her hair, ritually pouring the water in the Hogan near the door, and retires to reflect on her ceremony and her learning for a four more days.

The Mescalero Apache Girls' Puberty Ceremony occurs once a year for all young girls who have started their menses in the past year. The ceremony is an elaborate four-day public event, where male singers sing sixty-four different songs on each of the four nights. There is feasting, present giving, and dancing, and it is believed that this ceremony insures survival of the people. The four-day public ceremony is followed by a four-day private ceremony.

The first menstrual flow of Apache girls is met with an eight-day ceremony where the girl is honored by the people as a temporary manifestation of the female deity Isanaklesh. It is a proud day for the family, who recognizes the divinity now present in the power for bringing forth life. The girl is placed in her own tipi before dawn and carefully bathed and dressed for the ceremony. Her sponsor reminds her of how good it feels to be cared for, so that the girl will learn to care for others. This instilling of the idea that one must care for oneself well in order to know how to care well for others is a beautiful and meaningful inspiration that engenders true abilities to care for others as oneself.

Meanwhile, the girl's male kin construct a sacred tipi on ceremonial grounds. From there the power of the ceremonial songs will go out to all the people on Earth. The ceremony's songs, sacred narratives, and images combine for a powerful imprint of the deity on both the girl and her attending relatives and friends. For four days the girl allows only close relatives, friends, or those who wish to be blessed to her tipi. At night male dancers appear to bless her. The ceremony celebrates the transformation of adolescence into womanhood. Then for four more days the girl secludes herself to reflect on her ritual experience. There is a feast following the last day of the ceremony.

Blood rituals also mark the end of menses flow. Female companions of Tiwi women of Melville Island in Australia paint a red strip down the front of her body, symbolizing a snake. She is then led to another camp where her male relatives, and her future husband wait for her. A ceremonial spear is briefly placed between her legs and then presented to her intended husband, who hugs the spear calling it "wife." The girl's father places a palm tree upright in the ground and an elaborate game begins where the girl runs from her intended until he catches her. The husband-to-be and his brothers dance around her and women wash her, repaint her, and place feathered ornaments on her. She is then presented to her husband, but they are not allowed to talk to each other and she sleeps on the opposite side of the fire from him. The next morning the husband paints his wife, they may talk to each other, and wedded life begins.

Cherokee women follow a ritual at the end of every menses, ritually plunging seven times in running water and changing their clothes before going home. This plunge in running water removes anything that might harm their community and brings to them what they need to take back to their community. The Cherokee Plunge, used this way, is an extension of a purification ritual followed by both men and women as daily morning practice of offering to the river anything that they may be carrying emotionally that brings noxious energy to the day and to the community.

North American indigenous women have held rituals for every menses and for every birth. Ogala girls wrap up their first menstrual flow and put it in a tree to give them good influences throughout their lives. Zuni women perform ceremonies to celebrate the sex of their babies: A large seed-filled gourd is placed over a girl baby with prayers that her sexual parts grow large and her fruit abundant. A boy baby's penis is sprinkled with water with prayers that it remain small, implying that women's life-bearing capacity is immense in comparison to that of men. The act of hair brushing, viewed as an act of purification following first menses, exists today as a female ritual that has lost its original meaning.

Today few blood rituals designed by and for women exist in the modern world. In some cultures of today, it is the men who proclaim what is to be done with bleeding women, according to their religion or beliefs. Islamic women are secluded during menses, according to Islamic instructions that have ritualistic overtones derived from the Qu'ran. Until they have ceased menstruating and purified themselves, women are not allowed to participate in public worship. Orthadox Jewish women follow the same purification laws.

Sadly, in America, there are no rituals for menstruating girls or women, and the entire affair is treated as a scientific chemical change or something to be ignored or dismissed as interfering with normal progress. The modern world could learn much from the community blood rituals of the Dine, for it teaches respect as well as how to care for ourselves in order to care well for others.

Western Christian culture has offered us two diametrically opposite ways of being in the world, neither of which is balanced. Patriarchal values have taught us to look out for number one (ourselves at the expense of everyone else.) Christianity has taught us to sacrifice ourselves for the good of others, because "we are all sinners, and as such, are unworthy."

Children are confused in a world that offers a choice of selfish taking and altruistic giving, with no instructions on the relationship between the two. Somewhere between family of origin teachings and cultural values, each person decides how they are going to operate in the world. Those who choose (either consciously or from survival needs) to be caregivers would benefit greatly from learning to care for themselves before they offer care to others, but there is no training for this. There are thousands of articles and workshops offered to teach burned out caregivers the art of caring for themselves, but unfortunately, lifetime habits and ideas are difficult to change.

The dichotomy of values in Western culture, with the split defining of people who focus on selfishness ("me first" and "looking out for number one") and the caregivers, who have realized more deeply that we are all connected, causes a deep rift between people. Because there is little training on how to care for ourselves (as opposed to selfishly looking out *only* for ourselves), there is a true lack of balance between caring for ourselves and offering care to others. Caregivers suffer greatly in our culture from an inability to give the same loving care to themselves as they offer to everybody else.

A return to meaningful rituals surrounding the cycles of our lives would honor the return of the feminine, where everything is respected as part of the whole.

CONTRIBUTOR CONTACT INFORMATION

Ann DiSalvo
www.anndisalvo.com

May Jo Wootten
jwootten@indra.com

Donna Hertz
donnahertz@mac.com

Silvia Trujillo
silviastudio1@hotmail.com

Paula Fong
prfong@cpros.com

Meredith Killmer Hanson
meredithkhanson@yahoo.com

Laura Hurst
lauhurst@gmail.com

Windsong Dianne Martin
www.windsongmekani.com

Christer S. Rowan
www.rowandesign.com

REFERENCES

Achterberg, J. (1991). Woman as healer. Boston: Shambala.

Allen, P.G. (1986). The sacred hoop: Recovering the feminine in American Indian Traditions. Boston: Bacon Press.

Baker, R. (Ed.) (1980). The mystery of migration. New York: Viking Press.

Bettelheim, B. (1955). Symbolic wounds: Puberty rites and the envious male. New York, NY: Collier Books.

Briffault, R. (1927). The mothers. New York, NY:MacMillan.

Buckley, T. and Gottlieb, A. (1988). Blood magic: The anthropology of menstruation. Berkeley, CA: University of California Press.

Campbell, J. (1970). Myths, dreams, and religion. New York: E.P.Dutton & Co.

Capra, F. (1996). The web of life. New York: Doubleday.

Conrad, E. (2007). Life on land. Berkeley, CA: North Atlantic Books.

Coveney, P. & Highfield, R. (1990). The arrow of time. New York: Ballantine Books.

Csikszentmihalyi, M. (1990). Flow: The psychology of optimal experience. New York: Harper Perennial.

Delaney, J. (1976). The curse: A cultural history of menstruation. New York, NY: E.P. Dutton and Company.

Eliade, M. (1954). The myth of the eternal return. Princeton: Princeton University Press.

Feinstein, D. and Krippner, S. (1997). The mythic path: discovering the guiding star. New York: Jeremy Tarcher

Flinders, C. (2003). Rebalancing the world: why women belong and men compete and how to restore the ancient equilibrium. New York: Harper-Collins.

Ford, G. (1996). Listening to your hormones. Rocklin, CA: Prima Publishing.

Frazer, J.G. (1963). The golden bough: A study in magic and religion. New York, NY: MacMillan.

Frisbie, C.J. (1967). Kinaalda: A study of the Navaho girl's puberty ceremony. Salt Lake City: University of Utah Press.

Gardner, H. (1993). Creating minds. New York: Harper-Collins.

Gardner, R. (2004). Experimenting with water. Dover Publications.

George, D. (1992). Mysteries of the dark moon. San Francisco, CA: Harper Collins Publishers.

Gilligan, C. (1982). In a different voice: Psychological theory and women's development. Cambridge, MA: Harvard University Press.

Goldbeter, A. (1996). Biochemical oscillations and cellular rhythms. Cambridge, MA: Cambridge University Press.

Golub, S. (1985). Lifting the Curse of Menstruation. New York, NY: Harrington Park Press.

Gould, S.J. (1987). Time's arrow, time's cycle. Cambridge, MA: Harvard University Press.

Grahn, J. (1993). Blood, bread, and roses: How menstruation created the world. Boston, MA: Beacon Press.

Hales, D. (1999). Just like a woman: how gender science is redefining what makes us female. New York: Bantam.

Hobson, J.A. (1977). The dreaming brain. New York: Basic Books.

Knight, C. (1991). Blood relations: menstruation and the origins of culture. New Haven, CT: Yale University Press.

Kornfield, J. (1993). A path with heart. New York: Bantam Books.

Krippner, S. (2009.) Creativity and dreams. In, M. Runco and S. Pritzker (Eds.), Encyclopedia of creativity. San Diego: Academic Press.

Krippner, S. (2002). Extraordinary dreams and how to work with them. New York: State University of New York Press.

Madden, C.C. (1997). A room of her own. New York: Clarkson Potter Publishers.

Marks, W. (2001). The holy order of water. Herndon, VA: Bell Pond Books.

May, R. (1975). The Courage to Create. New York: Bantum Books.

Neuman, E. (1963). The great mother. Princeton, NJ: Princeton University Press.

Northrup, C. (2010). Women's bodies, women's wisdom: Creating physical and motional health and healing. New York, NY: Bantam Books.

Ogden, G. (2006). The heart and soul of sex. Boston: Trumpeter Books.

Orleane (RS) and Smith (CB) (2010). Conversations with Laarkmaa: A Pleiadian View of the New Reality. Bloomington, Indiana: AuthorHouse.

Orleane, R. (2001). Empowerment of women through sacred menstrual customs: effects of separate sleeping during menses on creativity, dreaming, relationships, and spirituality. San Francisco: Saybrook University.

Owen, L. (1993). Her blood is gold: Celebrating the power of menstruation. San Francisco, CA: Harper Collins.

Paper, J. (1997). Through the Earth darkly: Female spirituality in comparative perspective. New York, NY: Continum Press.

Parker, K.L. (Ed.). (1993). Wise women of the dreamtime. Rochester, VT: Inner Traditions International.

Perdue, T. (1998). Cherokee women: Gender and culture change, 1700-1835. Lincoln, NE: University of Nebraska Press.

Maya art. New York, NY: George Braziller, Inc.

Pert, C.B. (1997). Molecules of emotion. New York: Schribner.

Rako, S. (1996). The hormone of desire. New York: Harmony Books.

Runco, M. and Richards, R. (Eds.) (2009). Eminent creativity, everyday creativity, and health. Greenwich, CT: Ablex Publishing.

St. Pierre, M. and Long Soldier, T. (1995). Walking in the sacred manner: healers, dreamers, and pipe carriers-medicine women of the plains Indians. New York: Touchstone Press.

Sichel, D. and Driscoll, J. (1999). Women's moods. New York: William Morrow and Company.

Schwartz, M.T. Molded in the image of Changing Woman. Tucson, AZ: University of Arizona Press.

Schwenk, T. (1998). Sensitive chaos. Hernon, VA: Steiner Books.

Shuttle, P. and Redgrove, P. (1988). The wise wound: The myths, realities, and meanings of menstruation. New York, NY: Bantam Books.

St. Pierre, M. and Long Soldier, T. (1995). Walking in the sacred manner: Healers, dreamers, and pipe carriers-medicine women of the Plains Indians. New York, NY: Touchstone Press.

Steiner, F. (1954). Taboo. Harmondsworth: Penguin.

The Bible, Ecclesiastes.

The Encyclopedia Britannica: A dictionary of arts, science, literature & general information, (11th Ed.) 21. Cambridge, England: University Press.

Thoreau, H. (2009). Civil disobedience. New York: Classic Books America.

Vliet, E.L. (1995). Screaming to be heard. New York: M. Evans and Company.

Walker, B. (1983). The woman's encyclopedia of myths and secrets. San Francisco: Harper Collins.

Williamson, M. (1993). A woman's worth. New York: Ballantine.

ACKNOWLEDGMENTS

My first and most important thanks go to my heartmate, Cullen Baird Smith, who has kissed me alive and stood beside me through every challenge. I waited a long time for you! Thank you seeing me, for believing in me, appreciating me, sharing the gift of yourself with me, and for being my full partner in every sense of the word. What a joy to share my life with you!

Thanks to my creative mother, Jo Wootten, for telling me I could do anything if I reached for the stars and for loving me enough to grant me space to fly. Thanks to my real dad, Bob Finlay, for his ever present love.

Thanks to the late Anne Wootten Squires and my own Angels, Guides, Interdimensional Friends, and Spirit Teachers for beautiful and meaningful guidance and lessons along the way.

Thanks to Luzie and Bob Mason, Isabelle Murphy, and Billie Shea for always believing in me, supporting me, and laughing and crying with me. Special thanks to Rebecca Gretz, Genevieve Hangen, Wanda and Herb Blumenthal, Lora and Richard Dart, who love me as I am, share their insights on life, and listen to mine. Thank you, Lora, your valuable suggestions in the early version of this book. Thank you, Richard, for shared silences and long walks in Nature, which grounded me. Thank you Jewell and Kent Noonan for laughter, shared worldview, and the unparalleled acceptance and love found in true friendship.

Thanks to family members Bonnie Webb, Susan Deason, and Daniell Hamby for a shared sense of humor and support in negotiating our mutual family.

I thank Saybrook University for supporting not only my research, but also me as a person. Special thanks to Stan Krippner, Ruth Richards, Donald Rothberg, and Jeanne Achterberg, enlightened mentors with real heart. I also thank Greg Brack and the late Dave Danskin for early mentoring and encouraging me to think creatively. I thank Emilie Conrad, whose wisdom of the body is immense. What she knows, we all should know.

Thank you to all the women who provided art for this book. Special thanks to Christer Rowan, who provided professional integrity and creative solutions to all my emergency predicaments within the field of publishing. He is a true human being.

I am deeply grateful to the unnamed women who shared the most intimate explorations of their own journeys through Nature's gift as part of my research and to the indigenous elders who shared with me their understandings of sacred women's wisdom. Most of the ideas presented here are my own, but the background has been gathered from multiple sources. I acknowledge all who contributed to my knowledge base and understanding through their own ideas, studies, and gathering of information. For a detailed list of all sources, please see the extended Bibliography in my research dissertation.

In order to help women know that we *always* have a choice, I wish to acknowledge the gifts that came as hard lessons from being in two difficult, if not impossible, marriages. Through those men's persistent attempts to define (wrongly) who I was, I learned to trust my own knowing and to stand up for myself. Because they thought that they could own my spirit, I fled, proving that only *I* own my own soul.

I acknowledge the wisdom of Nature and express my thanks for all the ways that I am, indeed, part of Her. For Life, Beauty, Changeability, Spirituality, Flow, Connection, Joy, Love, and the Power of the Present Moment, I am grateful.